The Magical Sodium, Calcium, And Magnesium

"Create A Powerful Alkaline Body Using These Minerals"

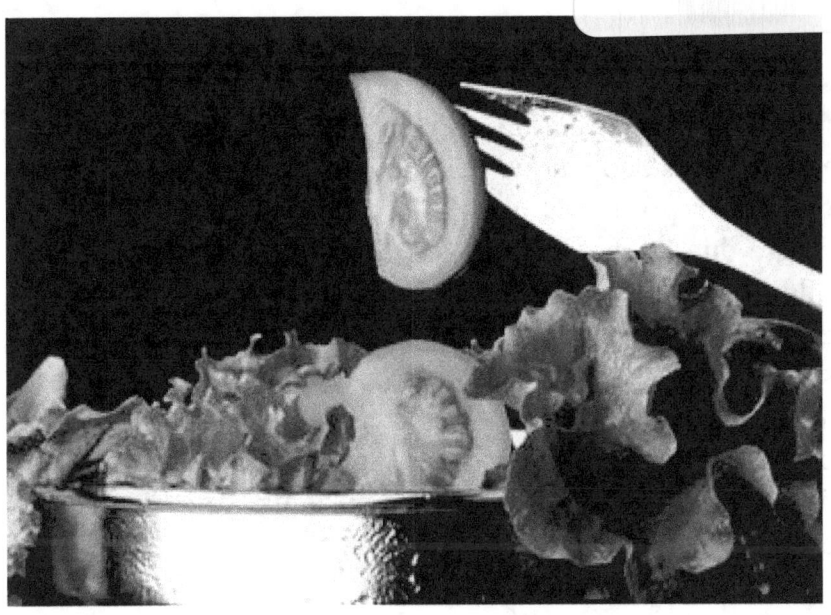

By Rudy S Silva, Natural Nutritionist

TABLE OF CONTENTS

Section 1: Sodium

Chapter 1: Introduction

"Sodium is considered the Youth Element, since in the right proportions in your body, it will keep you young"

Your body has amazing ways that it can prolong your life. Many people and scientist look at the body from a chemical view point, but in fact it is an electrical body. In his book, The Philosopher's Stone, Michiio Kushi recounts how he performed an experiment in his laboratory where he transmuted sodium, $Na+$ into Potassium, $K+$. Having the right sodium in your body can provide transmutation when you need it.

In this Kindle e-book you will discover why you should be concerned about sodium foods and your sodium diet and how this is related to potassium. In the end, it's all about how you can have the best health by minimizing any health problems that can arise from having an imbalance of sodium with respect with other minerals.

Sodium, chloride, and potassium, calcium, magnesium and phosphorus are a few of the critical electrolytes or ions in your body. Sodium is a positive charged electrolyte that resides mostly outside of your body cells.

Sodium stands number one in importance in your body. Ninety percent of the sodium ions, $Na+$, that exist in the fluids outside of your cells are sodium. It is sodium that attracts fluids and water into the outer cellular area and maintains the balance of these fluids throughout your body.

Sodium is an alkaline mineral that has a positive charge like potassium that neutralizes acids, whereas potassium helps to drain acids out of the body. The chemical symbol for sodium ions is Na+ and for potassium it is K+. This indicates that Na lacks an electron in its outer orbit and will readily accept an electron so that it can be balanced electrically.

Since Chloride has one extra electron in its outer electron orbit, it can contribute this electron to sodium. The result is that sodium and chloride have an affinity for each other and that is why you see NaCl as a product better known as table salt. You have approximately 3 ounces of sodium in your body.

In the presence of water, NaCl will dissociate into the ions Na+ and Cl-. When you eat food that contain sodium, your stomach acid will break down your food and in the process release the sodium in the food to form Na+. It is in this form that your body uses Na+ and it is found though out your body eliminating acid. It also serves to create electrical potentials across cell membranes, small littler batteries that help to move nutrients across cell walls.

Many diseases are caused because people lack organic sodium, not table salt, in their diet and are deficient in it in their body liquids. Sodium is called the Youth Element, because if you always have the right amount in your body, you will be limber, pliable, and active. All athletic activities and active hobbies require your body to have plenty of sodium.

Organic Sodium

The difference between organic sodium and inorganic sodium, table salt, is organic sodium is found only in fruits and vegetables. It is alive and has electric magnetic energy and frequencies that your body uses to energizing itself. But inorganic sodium found in table salt and in many other processed foods and is considered dead food. Table salt is not alive and is not the correct sodium that the body needs for good health, but your body will still use it as a substitute when you lack organic salt.

Inorganic Sodium

Salt, sodium chloride, is not a food and is considered inorganic sodium. All inorganic substances are harmful to your body. Salt is crystal found in natural deep in the earth. It's mined and brought up to the surface where it is sorted and purified into various sizes. When it is dissolved by forcing water deep into the earth it is called Brine.

Salt is used in many industries. It is used in thousands of applications from meat packers, food to leather processors. It is used to manufacture glass, soap, and paper. It is used in water, to build roads, refine metals, and make ice cream. It is not a food, but it is used as a seasoning in many foods.

Sodium In Your Body

Like calcium and potassium, sodium has many functions throughout your body and is stored throughout your body, for emergencies. It keeps calcium and magnesium in solution and prevents them from precipitating. It is active in the blood, lymph, lymph nodes, stomach, colon, cells, tissues, and wherever acid is formed in your body.

Sodium maintains the proper extracellular fluid volume, liquid outside cells, since it attracts water. If you have edema, excess water in your body, or high blood pressure, you need to back off on eating salt. When you don't have enough salt, you will lack water in your body. This has a dramatic effect on your blood pressure, since it will cause low blood pressure.

Sodium with the help of potassium and chloride also helps transit impulses in nerve and muscle fibers. All along nerve fibers sodium exists creating an electric voltage across the nerve membranes, so that nerve impulses can travel to the various locations in your body.

Sodium is lost from your body in hot humid weather and when you do hard physical work. Sauna baths, fevers, sweating, passion, extreme excitement also causes sodium loss. Self-abuse and self-hatred also causes loss of sodium. You will also lose sodium when you have an acid body. Sodium is used to neutralize acids and is used up when you have an excess to neutralize.

Sodium also maintains your cell permeability. It moves into your cells and out of your cells as it transports sugars and amino acids into your cells. It is involved in muscle contractions.

Sodium is also found in the blood and there it functions to keep other mineral soluble, so that they do not precipitate out to form deposits. It helps to move carbon dioxide out of your body and is involved in the production of HCL acid in your stomach. It provides a protective layer in your stomach so that HCL does not create ulcers in your stomach lining.

A deficiency in sodium can also result in decreased iron chemical activity. Sodium is needed so that your body can use iron.

Daily Sodium Requirements

You only need around 500 milligrams of sodium per day, but most people who do not watch their salt use get around 4400 to 8800 milligram per day. Since sodium attracts water, eating high levels of sodium each day usually leads to high blood pressure due to extra water in the blood vessels.

Sodium Bicarbonate

Sodium bicarbonate, $NaHCO_3$, or sodium hydrogen carbonate is the common baking soda and many people know this better as Alka-Seltzer. You can use sodium bicarbonate for stomach indigestion for a short time. However, using it long term to alleviate your stomach problems can result in side effects. It is also used to make your blood or urine less acidic.

When sodium bicarbonate is used long term, the bicarbonate part of this chemical, HCO3, is readily absorbed into the body causing a pH change in your body. This result in a condition called Systemic Alkalosis.

Systemic Alkalosis is a condition where excess bicarbonate ions are in your tissue causing the pH to exceed 7.4. This is the opposite of having an acid body and is a condition where there is an excess of alkaline ions throughout your body. Normally the kidneys will excrete the excess bicarbonate, but there are a few conditions that prevent the kidney from removing the excess bicarbonate, which then leads to Systemic Alkalosis.

One of the effects of alkalosis is an excess of sodium in your body, which comes from the sodium bicarbonate and puts your body's pH out of balance. When you have an excess of sodium in your body, it can lead to a variety of various body conditions – edema, high blood pressure, or cell malfunction.

Some of the side effects of prolong use of sodium bicarbonate, which come from the bicarbonate are:

- severe headache or nausea
- loss of appetite
- irritability or weakness
- frequent urge to urinate
- swelling of legs for feet
- dark or bloody stools
- Blood in urine

Taking sodium bicarbonate pills to relieve an acid body is not recommended. This compound should not be used for medical purposes without direction from a doctor.

Chapter 2: Activities Of Sodium In Your Body

Organic Sodium helps to keep calcium in solution. When your body lacks sodium, calcium will precipitate from solution and create calcium crystals in different parts of your body. When you eat table salt, your body removes calcium from your body and excretes it in your urine.

What you eat and absorb will determine what amount of sodium your body has. The actual sodium requirement of each person differs based on age and size. You need less than 3 grams of sodium daily, but the average American diet provide around 6 gram. It's the kidneys that help to keep excess sodium out of your body, by excreting it in your urine. Other parts of your body will also eliminate sodium – skin, colon, and all liquid discharges.

In his book, Dr. Colgan, Michael, Optimum Sports Nutrition, New York, Advanced Research Press, 1993 say,

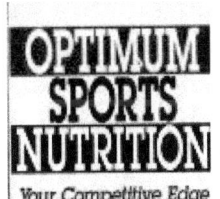

"From all the ads for electrolyte replacement drinks for use during and after exercise, you would think that athletes need more sodium. Except for some ultra-distance athletes (Ironman length triathlons, 100-mile running races) that's just promotional flapdoodle. The human body conserves its electrolytes."

Dr Colgan says that after exercise you don't need electrolytes or sodium because you lose water during exercise by sweating but your body keeps the electrolytes in your body. You only need to drink water, because now your water to electrolytes is out of balance.

In the beginning of any exercise, you lose some sodium in your sweat, but as you continue your exercise or sport, your body at some point starts to conserve your sodium. The result is that you don't lose much sodium as has been previous thought by many doctors, sports people or people. You don't need those sports drinks that say brings your electrolytes back to normal, when you are working or playing hard.

Sodium and water go together. Sodium attracts water. So if your sodium intake increases and is reflected as an increase sodium in your body, your body will retain more water. The more sodium you have in your body the more water you need to balance this sodium.

When you get thirsty, the posterior pituitary gland will release an anti-diuretic hormone, so that your kidney does not excrete too much water to your bladder. This will help you to maintain the water you have in your body.

When your body sodium decreases, your thirst disappears, the anti-diuretic hormone is suppressed, and the kidney excretes more liquid into your bladder. The result is your body starts to excrete the excess water.

In some cases, you can have an excess of sodium in your body. People who are overweight should decrease their intake of sodium, since sodium attracts water and can add body weight.

Excess sodium has been also associated with a higher risk of cancer, since it upsets the sodium potassium balance. People who eat a diet of high salted foods such as fish, pork, or dried meat upset the sodium potassium balance. The sodium potassium balance is required, since it is these two elements that maintain the right electrical voltage across your body cells. When this voltage is upset, it leads to disease.

What Sodium Does In Your Body

As was mention, one of the key functions of sodium is to maintain your water balance throughout your body and in this process it helps to keep your cells healthy. It is also involved in neutralizing acid molecules that accumulate in your body, from the food you eat, the polluted air you breathe, the negative thoughts you have, or the bad water you drink.

How Sodium Keeps Cells Functioning

Understanding one portion of how your cells work through the use of sodium and potassium is an important step in knowing why you should strive to eat the right sodium foods and to not eat an excess of table salt.

Sodium is found outside and inside of your cells. You have 1000 mg of sodium your body. Fifty percent of that is in your extracellular fluid, outside of your cells, 10% inside of your cells, and 40% in your bones. Typically there are 7% sodium ions inside your cells and 93% outside your cells. Your size and age determine how much sodium your body needs. What you eat and how you absorb your food will determine how much sodium goes into your body.

Typically, your body needs around 200mg to 500 mg of sodium daily, but it has been found that people intake up to 6000 mg daily. If you have normal functioning kidneys, the amount of sodium maintained in your body is constant. The kidneys will excrete excess sodium from your body. Sodium is also excreted in feces and sweat

In your body sodium and water go together. If you eat too much sodium the water in your body will increase. If you eat less sodium, the amount of water held in the extracellular fluids will decrease.

Your body controls the amount of water you maintain in your body by a diuretic and anti-diuretic hormone that is release to pass more water out your kidney as urine or to not pass water out of your body. When your sodium level increases, your body makes you thirsty so you will drink more water.

Sodium Potassium Pump

Sodium and potassium ions exist outside your cells, extracellular liquid, and inside your cells, intracellular liquid. In the cell, there is around 7% sodium and 92% potassium. Outside the cell there is the opposite, 93% sodium and 8% potassium. These are the percentage that should be maintained for good cellular function. Naturally, sodium tends to diffuse into the cell while potassium tends to diffuse out of the cell.

The sodium-potassium pump is embedded in the cell membrane and opens to move sodium or potassium ions back and forth across from outside to inside or from inside to outside the cells. This is done to keep a certain voltage across the cell membrane. This potential allows sugar or glucose and amino acids to move into the cell using the sodium-potassium pump. As cells use up nutrients brought in, toxic matter is created. This toxic matter is then transported out of the cell using the sodium-potassium pump.

Go to the following link to view sodium pump process.

http://url2it.com/msrc
or
http://url2it.com/msrd

So now you can see the importance of maintain the proper levels of sodium in your body.

A diet rich in sodium provides the body with the sodium to neutralize acids in your kidney and liver. Sodium works to eliminate acetic, buturic, lactic and other fatty acids, which are derived from starchy foods, lard, margarine, potatoes, oily nuts, and meats. These foods cause the precipitation of sodium and potassium and deplete them, if you continually eaten them.

When sodium is deficient, bad bacteria takes over your digestive tract. In the colon, sodium keeps the environment slightly alkaline to control the bad bacterial.

Sodium Deficiencies

Here are some of the symptoms you will have if you have a deficiency of body sodium:

Gout	cracking joints	excess mucus
Dull complexion	tendons stiff	bloating
Restless nerves	fatigue	constipation
Mental confusion	drowsiness	Frontal headache
Bad breath	Lack of saliva	white coated tongue

Because fruits and vegetables are naturally grown from soil, they pull minerals out of the ground and can be a great source of minerals like sodium for you. Because of these minerals and other nutrients, fruits and vegetables have amazing curative effects, when they are eaten raw.

If you have an acid body, like most people do, this is what is causing your illness. You need to move your acid body into an alkaline condition and sodium, calcium, magnesium, and other minerals can help you to do this. See chapter 13, so you can see how to make your body more alkaline.

Chapter 3: Detrimental Effects of Table Salt

Your body does not need table salt. But it does need sodium and chloride, which is found naturally in food. Your body stores sodium and has plenty, if you eat the right kind of food. When you have a poor diet or have a destructive lifestyle, you deplete your sodium.

There are many detrimental effects of eating too much table salt. However, these effects are not related to the sodium you get from the food you eat. This is because the sodium you get from natural food, which has not been cooked, is electrically charged and has energy associated with it. Table salt is a dead food and has no electrical charge associated with it.

Bone Density

When you eat salt, calcium is excreted from your body and this leads to lower bone density. Granted the amount of calcium lost is small, but over time it can be significant. If you drink coffee, then caffeine will cause you to lose a little bit more bone density.

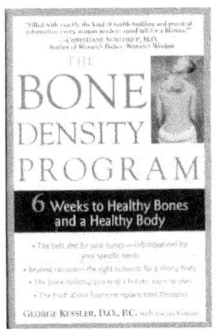

In his book, Kessler, George D.O., P.C. and Kapklein, Colleen, The Bone Density Program, New York, Ballantine Books, 2000, he points out that,

"As with high blood pressure, some people seem to be more sensitive to the effects of salt that others. But the group of sensitive people is large enough that everyone would be wise to use discretion when it comes to salt. Since you don't automatically know whether you are sensitive... Stay within the American Heart Association's guidelines (2,000 mg a day or less) to be safe."

Heart Disease and Cancer

Many studies have been done on how salt contributes to heart disease and cancer. It has been thought that high salt diets contribute to heart diseases.

But in Dr. Watts,L. David, Trace Elements and Other Essential Nutrients, Texas, 4th Writer;s B-L-O-C-K, 2003, he clarifies studies that point to chlorine as the major contributor to heart and cancer diseases.

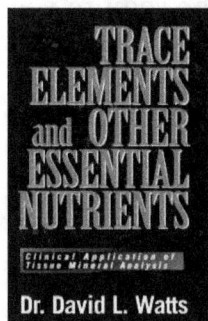

Dr. David L. Watts

"It now appears that the salt-hypertension link was overly exaggerated. In fact, stringent salt restriction is only necessary for a small segment of the affected population. Only about 10-15 percent may benefit from limiting salt intake. These are a group of individuals with high blood pressure who are classified as 'salt-sensitive.' More recent studies implicate chloride in the development of hypertension rather than sodium alone. Animal studies have shown that high amounts of sodium chloride can induce an elevation in blood pressure."

The actual cause of high blood pressure is not that clear cut, since many people with high blood pressure may have a number of mineral imbalances. Some people are sensitive to sodium and some to chloride and these sensitivities can cause various health issues.

Another factor involved in heart disease is the sodium to potassium ratio. Dr. Julian Whitaker, M.D. points out that most people have a ratio of twice as much sodium as potassium in the body. By changing this ratio, Dr. Whitaker claims you can protect yourself from heart and cancer. To do this you need to watch your salt intake and learn which foods give you more potassium and add them to your diet.

Excess salt has also been known as a stomach cancer threat. This is especially true when the sodium in salt combines with other carcinogens – barbecue smoke, grilled meat, sodium nitrides, or pesticides. Salt irritates the stomach, which increases the disposition of precancerous cell replication and powers chemical carcinogen to do more stomach damage. When your diet is low in fruits and vegetables, the results of a high salt diet are even more damaging.

Kidney Damage

When you eat salt, your body tries to get rid of it. It does this by making you thirsty. If you drink more water, your kidney will cause you to urinate more. This is how your body tries to get rid of the salt you eat.

Of all your body organs, your kidneys suffer the most when you eat salt. If you eat more salt than your kidneys can remove, your kidneys breakdown the salt and deposit it in various parts of your body, but mostly in your lower legs. Then your body tries to protect itself from this salt by bringing water to that area. This causes swelling in the legs and feet. This also causes puffy eyelids and bags underneath your eyes.

Fluid Retention and Sodium Restricted diet

In cases where excess sodium has been consumed and where the kidney has not expelled the excess, fluid retention disease starts to appear, if the excess sodium condition continues to exist. Fluid retention diseases are congestive heart failure and edema. Other excess sodium conditions are kidney failure, adrenal disease, and cirrhosis of the liver. Under these conditions, a sodium restricted diet is called for. Using the information in this kindle e-book provides you with a good start in restricting your use of table salt in your diet.

A diet rich in sodium provides the body with the sodium to neutralize acids in your kidney and liver. Sodium works to eliminate acetic, buturic, lactic and other fatty acids, which are derived from starchy foods, lard, margarine, potatoes, oily nuts, and meats. These foods cause the precipitation of sodium and potassium and deplete them, if you continually eaten them.

When sodium is deficient, bad bacteria takes over your digestive tract. In the colon, sodium keeps the environment slightly alkaline to control the bad bacterial.

Sodium Deficiencies

Here are some of the symptoms you will have if you have a deficiency of body sodium:

Gout	cracking joints	excess mucus
Dull complexion	tendons stiff	bloating
Restless nerves	fatigue	constipation
Mental confusion	drowsiness	Frontal headache
Bad breath	Lack of saliva	white coated tongue

Because fruits and vegetables are naturally grown from soil, they pull minerals out of the ground and can be a great source of minerals like sodium for you. Because of these minerals and other nutrients, fruits and vegetables have amazing curative effects, when they are eaten raw.

If you have acid body, like most people do, this is what is causing your illness. You need to move your acid body into an alkaline condition and sodium and other minerals can help you to do this.

CHAPTER 4: SODIUM DIET FOODS YOU MUST EAT

When joints start to get hard and painful to move, they lack nutrients or specific minerals. With arthritis, sodium is lacking, so sodium foods recommended are okra and celery, which are also available in tablets. Goat whey is another good source of sodium and can be purchased on the internet. To get more information on goat whey, just type this word into Google search.

Other fruits and vegetables that are high in sodium should also be eaten. Only fruits that are picked ripe should be eaten. If they are picked green and allowed to become ripe, they will not have as much sodium, since the sun helps to create the sodium in food.

Some people who have symptoms related to sodium deficiencies may recover quickly or may take a long time to benefit from the addition of sodium. It takes up to 3 months to replenish the sodium reserves in your body, when they are low. And this is providing you are eating an excess of fruits and vegetables.

Sodium and the stomach

The stomach is considered a sodium organ, since it stores sodium in its walls to prevent stomach acid from burning a hole in its tissue. As stomach HCl, hydrochloric acid, moves against your stomach walls, sodium neutralizes it, preventing it from damaging your stomach walls.

The sodium you eat first goes to the stomach walls and the excess goes to the joints. So if you have joint problems you most likely have stomach problems also.

Sodium Foods

Raw goat milk and goat whey are foods high in sodium. Black mission figs are also high in sodium.

Here is a broth that you can make to get extra sodium and potassium called Veal Joint Broth as described by Bernard Jensen, Ph.D.

"Use a clean, fresh, uncut veal joint and after washing in cold water, put into a large cooking pot: cover half with water and add the following vegetables and greens cut up finely:

Small stalk of celery

1 ½ cups apple peelings, ½ in thick

2 cups potato peeing, ½ in thick

½ cup chopped parsley

2 beets, grated

1 large parsnip

1 onion

½ cup okra

Simmer all ingredients for 4 or 5 hours: strain off liquid and discard solid ingredients. There should be 1 ½ quarts of liquid. Drink hot or cold and keep refrigerated."

These are the foods high in sodium:

Apples	kale	kelp	lentils
Dried apricots	asparagus	barley	raw milk
Beets	mustard greens	greens	beets
Red cabbage	okra	carrots	parsley
Celery	dried peas	cheeses	chickpeas
Red peppers	coconut	prunes	raisins
Collard	sesame	spinach	dates
Dulse	strawberries	egg yolks	sunflower
Figs	Swiss chard	turnips	goat milk
Artichokes	lemons	parsley	watercress

Every day you should be eating these various vegetables. You want to make sure you eat at least three highly colored vegetables with your lunch and dinner – bright green, red, orange, yellow, purple and so on. The more colors you can include in your meals the healthier you will be.

Minimize Your Use Of Salt

Since you have probably been using salt for a long time, you have become accustom to having a lot of salt in your food. You can use other ways to spice up your food, without using a lot of salt. Here are a few ways to do this.

Use herbs, spices, and culinary herbs

Use lemon or lime juice to flavor your food

Don't use salt in cooking nor have it on your table

Use butter that is salt free. Don't use margarine, since it has trans fatty acids or hydrogenated oils.

Most canned foods or processed foods are high in sodium. Look for those are low sodium or sodium free.

Choose breakfast cereals that are low in sodium

Fresh meat, poultry, fish are low in sodium. But avoid the processed meats.

Use low sodium soy sauce

Avoid teriyaki sauce and miso sauce, which are very high in sodium

Avoid boiling vegetable with salt added, vegetables will absorb the salt

Use these labels to determine how much sodium is in food you buy per serving.

Sodium – Free, contains less than five mg of sodium.

Very low sodium, contains less than 34 mg of sodium.

Low – sodium, has less than 141 mg of sodium.

Reduced – sodium, has 75% of sodium found in normal food.

Salt Replacement

You can completely eliminate the need to use salt in your food preparation or reduce its use to a very low amount. This is done by becoming familiar with spices and culinary herbs. By consistently using herbs and spices you get fantastic good taste and their therapeutically benefits. The best way to use herbs and spices is to read about their use in food and create a blend that you can use over and over.

Here are some spices to consider:

Basil – use in tomato sauces, soups, salads. Place a small amount in your palm then rub both hands to break the tiny flakes and let them fall into your soup.

Cloves – use with pumpkin and squash dishes or to spice up your rice and baked goods dishes.

Garlic – is part of the onion family and it should be used every day and in as many different dishes that you prepare.

Ginger – use it in cooking meat, stir fry, cookies, or cakes.

Paprika – use it to liven up chicken, mashed potatoes or broiled fish.

Red pepper powder – use it in soups, stews, sauces. You can use a variety of different pepper powders. Try the Eagle brand chili powder, which contains more than one type of chili pepper.

Rosemary – used to flavor chicken, turkey, and lamb.

Turmeric – use with curries.

You can get fresh herbs such as basil, dill, parsley, cilantro or mint. Put the dried herbs into your pot early in your cooking. For fresh herbs, wait until near the end of your cooking.

One of the ways to use herbs is to create a blend that you can add to your dishes as you cook them. You can create a blend for different types of dishes that you cook. Through experimenting with different herbs and spice you can make your own blends. Here are a couple of simple blends.

For Italian Dishes – use only the amount you need.

1 tablespoon of dried oregano
1 tablespoon dried basil
1 tablespoon of dried thyme

For **Mexican soups** add and taste

1 tablespoon of dried oregano

1 tablespoon of basil
1 tablespoon of chili powder
1 tablespoon of a variety of chili powders
1/2 tablespoon of cumin

A **general blend** would be like this

1 tablespoon of dried basil
2 teaspoons of celery seed
2 teaspoons of dried savory
1 teaspoon of dried thyme
1 teaspoon of dried marjoram

Sodium bicarbonate

Organic Sodium bicarbonate, $NaHCO_3$, contains sodium, hydrogen, carbon and oxygen and is also known as baking soda. Organic sodium bicarbonate is created in your body and is used when you have mucus congestions in the throat and bronchial areas. When you have these conditions, sodium foods are recommended. Bicarbonate is also called for to reduce gout, diabetic acid, subacid blood, and stomach mucus.

Saliva

Saliva is an alkaline substance, which is used to neutralize acids as they enter your mouth. It is composed of many different alkaline compounds, such as calcium, sodium, and magnesium phosphates, sodium and potassium chlorides, and sodium carbonate.

Sodium is involved in a variety of digestion processes as food goes into your mouth, stomach and small intestine.

Bile

Your bile that comes from your liver into your gallbladder consists of:

- Sodium carbonate
- Sodium phosphate
- Potassium chloride
- Sodium chloride
- Lecithin
- Sodium palmitate
- Sodium stearate
- Cholesterin
- Sodium taurocholate
- Sodium glycocholate
- Water

When your body doesn't have enough sodium, it will take it from your bile in the gallbladder and as sodium is depleted from the bile, cholesterol will precipitate causing gallstones.

Bile is necessary for you to have regular bowel movements, since it stimulates peristaltic colon action. When your liver is not putting out enough bile, you will have constipation. When you have enough bile your stool will be a light brown.

Hidden Salt

There are many processed foods that contain sodium chloride or inorganic salt. This is the type of salt that creates sickness, when consumed in excess. As you look at the various foods you buy, look at the nutritional label and buy only those foods that have less salt.

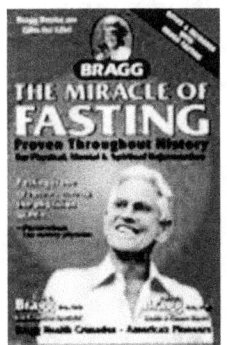

In his Bragg Health Series, N.D., PhD, Bragg, G., Paul and Bragg Patricia, N.D., PhD, The Miracle of Fasting, California, Health Science, they recall an incident that shows the deadly power of salt,

"The most dramatic wrongful death case against salt occurred in a Binghamton, New York hospital, where a number of babies died when salt was inadvertently used in their formula. An overdose of salt can kill a baby quickly. The body needs natural, organic sodium – not table salt, an inorganic chemical. You can obtain natural sodium which Mother Nature provides in organic form in celery, beets, carrots, potatoes, soybeans, turnips sea vegetation, seaweed, kelp, watercress, etc. and many other natural healthy foods. Remember, only organic minerals can be utilized by your body's living cells."

The amount of organic sodium you need per day is up to 500mg. But because there is hidden salt in most processed foods and by your use of table salt, you probable consume from 500 to 6000 mg per day.

Here are a few of the foods with hidden salt to look out for:

- ❖ Cured meats – bacon, hot dogs, sliced processed meats, sausages
- ❖ Canned soups, canned tuna, prepared pancakes
- ❖ TV dinners
- ❖ Regular soy sauce
- ❖ Tomato sauces
- ❖ All packaged foods

Sodium in your drinking water

There is also sodium in the bottled water that you drink. The amount it has is based on the brand. Some bottled water has very little and others have up to 200 mg or more. If you are on a strict sodium diet, then you need to know which bottled water has less sodium.

Most bottle water companies put sodium into their water so that it tastes better. But, some do not and just allow what is in the water to exist. Companies that produce low –salt or no-salt water must list the sodium contain in their bottles.

Water that is labeled Natural Spring Water has sodium but this type of water has the lowest sodium content as compared to other bottled water. If you drink distilled water then there is no sodium in this type of water.

Sodium Compounds Which Attack Your Immune System

Sodium has the ability to form many compound inside and outside your body. Many food suppliers tend to put a variety of sodium compounds in your food to make it taste better or to have a better consistency. These compounds tend to erode cells and tissue creating clumps of deadly free radicals. The result of this is that they use up a lot of your antioxidants that you need elsewhere in your body.

Here is a list of these sodium compounds that you want to avoid. Read the labels on the food you buy and check that the food you buy is free of these compounds.

Salt, sodium chloride – is a destructive compound, which you should eat less of. Get your sodium by eating more sodium foods.

Baking powder – used in various baking products.

Baking soda, sodium bicarbonate – used to relieve various stomach issues.

Brine, table salt or water – used in foods to control growth of bacteria and in cleaning fruits and vegetables, in freezing or canning certain foods, and for flavoring corned beef, pickles, sauerkraut, French fries.

Disodium phosphate – used in quick cooking cereals or processed cheeses.

Monosodium glutamate - comes in many different brands, used in packaged or frozen foods.

Sodium alginate – used in some chocolate milks and ice cream

Sodium benzoate – used as a preservative in sauces and salad dressings.

Sodium hydroxide – used to soften olives, hominy and some fruits and vegetables.

Sodium propionate – used in pasteurized cheeses, some breads and cakes to inhibit mold.

Sodium sulfite – used to bleach fruits for artificial colors, such as cherries, dried fruit.

Sodium nitrate or sodium nitrite – a dangerous preservative that is used on meat, which is considered carcinogen, cancer forming.

Sodium citrate – a chemical used in food that is harmful to your health.

Sodium dioctyl sulfate, Colace, – used as a lubricant in laxative products and can be habit forming

Chapter 5: Salt Bath Curative Effects

External Use Of Salt

Eating sodium is not the only way to get it into your body. It can be used externally as a natural remedy. Salt can be used in many ways to heal and detoxify your body. In combination with water, salt can be applied externally and have a positive effect on your body's pH and health. It is recommended that you use coarse salt or sea salt for your footbath, tub bath, or massage.

The types of salts below can be found by searching on Google. Type in coarse salt and get a variety of sites that sell this type of salt and many others that you can use for your bath.

Here some of the different types of salts you can use:

- ❖ Celtic sea salt
- ❖ Himalayan Crystal Salt, food grade
- ❖ Coarse sea salt
- ❖ Dead Sea Bath Salt -
- ❖ Epson Salt
- ❖ Atlantic Sea Bath Salt

Epson salt is used to create strong perspiration. It is a muscle relaxer and should not be used, if you are not in good health. The dead sea salt can help you, if you have had an injury.

What makes these salts great is that you not only have regular salt, $NaCl2$, but they contain many other mineral salts – magnesium and potassium salts. Not all salts have the same minerals, so you have to check the specifications. Using salts that have a variety of minerals is a great way to get curative effects, when they are used as massage or bath.

Salt Massage Bath

You will want to do a salt massage bath, when you want to stop an oncoming cold, relieve gout pain, restore blood and lymph circulation, overcome sluggishness, and to clean your skin of dirt and dead skin.

This type of massage will improve your mood and reduce your stress as the friction of the salt goes over your skin. It acts as a skin and body stimulant, by increasing blood circulation. If you have a mild case of depression this will help you.

Here's how to do it. Use plain coarse salt, sea salt, or many of the other salts.

Create a slushy salt paste with warm water. You can sit in the tub or shower and pour some salt and water into your hands and create a paste. Apply this paste all over your body from shoulders to feet in a slow circular motion. If you want you can place your feet in hot water as you massage your body. Do the massage only for a few minutes.

After your massage, wash off salt with a gentle shower of slightly warm water and rub your skin with a sponge to remove the salt and stimulate your skin.

If you have any open cuts do not do the salt massage in those areas. Also if you have skin lesions or skin inflammation, do not do the massage.

Complete immersion Salt Bath

Use a salt bath when you need to relax. If you have been sitting in your chair all day and have had a lot anxiety then a salt bath will help you release tension. If you need to clean your skin of dirt or dead skin, a salt bath will help you do this. Women in menopause will benefit for a salt bath.

Here how to do it.

In a tub of warm water put 1 to 2 cups of salt crystals. The more cups you use, the more you will perspire. To simulate sea water you can use 5 pounds of coarse salt and this will act as a mild tonic on your body. You can use water at 65 to 75 F for your bath but stay in the bath for 2 minutes or so. With warmer water you can stay in the bath for up to 15 minutes. Finish your bath with a warm shower and rub your body with a sponge or cloth.

Chapter 6: The Secrets of Sodium

The difference between organic sodium and inorganic sodium is critical to understand and apply. Organic sodium is only found in natural produce and is available to you when you eat fresh produce. When this produce is stored and sprayed for storage and transport, it loses is potential to provide you with the best sodium and other minerals.

Your body only uses organic sodium because it has electrical energy in the form of ions and frequency. The frequency come from its color and it is this energy that the cells use to provide you with the energy you need to run your body.

Whereas inorganic sodium is in table salt and this is the type of sodium that you find in most grocery store package products. When you eat table salt your body tries to get rid of it. This is why sodium attracts so much water. Through water, your body can eliminate this salt in your urine.

But if you eat too much salt, your kidneys are overwhelmed and can't get rid of all of it. So, it stores this salt in different parts of your body. The result is that you gain weight and develop sickness. Excess body water creates edema. In your cells excess water will appear and now the electrical potential that is between outside and the inside your cell is changed and your cell will not work properly.

Organic sodium is used throughout your body and it first goes to your stomach walls where it is stored to prevent the high stomach acid from burning a hole in your stomach - stomach ulcers. Then it is used to keep your joints from drying out by attracting water to the area needed. Since sodium is part of the Potassium – Sodium Pump, the amount of sodium is closely regulated by your body so that you don't have an excess. Natural food has the proper ratio of potassium and sodium the body needs.

An excess of sodium attracts water and excess water will cause your body cells to function less efficiently. When you are deficient in sodium you will have a variety of symptoms and illnesses that will start to develop. You can maintain adequate supply of sodium in your body, by eating raw fruits and vegetables and goat whey.

Most likely, you will not have an excess of salt, unless you eat a lot of salty meats and use plenty of salt with your meals. Since your body uses sodium to reduce acids in your body, sodium is used up quickly and your sodium reserves can become depleted.

Most people have acid bodies and that's one reason they have various illnesses. What this means is that they are deficient in organic sodium and they are not able to neutralize all of the acid that is created in their body from the acid foods that they eat. Acid foods like meat, potatoes, butter, carbohydrates need to be balanced with alkaline foods like fruits and vegetables. To understand how to change an acid body to an alkaline body check my Kindle e-book called, "Secret Diet And Nutrition (Nutrition Tips: Alkaline Body).

Here is something for you to do to get more natural sodium into your body. Go to the internet and look up goat milk and goat whey. Read about the benefits you can get by using these products. Then the next time you go to a health food store see if they have raw goat milk or goat whey.

They might have raw goat milk depending on what state you live in and mostly likely you can only find goat whey on the internet as "whex." Goat milk is an alkaline food and has a lot of sodium. Even raw cow's milk is alkaline, but when it is pasteurized or homogenized it becomes an acid food.

Chapter 7: Choosing The Best Sodium Foods

Here is a more comprehensive list of food and the amount of sodium they contain. This is based on 3 1/2 cups of the food. This list is to give you an idea of the amount of sodium in both processed foods and fruits and vegetables. You should pick those foods that are more natural and that are not processed, which have the highest sodium value. Those foods with high potassium value are also important.

Meat and Poultry*	Portion	Sodium (mg.)	Potassium (mg.)
Bacon	1 strip (1 oz.)	71	16
Beef			
Corned Beef(canned)	3 slices	803	51
Hamburger	¼ lb.	41	382
Pot Roast (rump)	¼ lb.	43	309
Sirloin Steak	½ lb.	57	545
Chicken (broiler)	3\12 oz.	78	320
Duck	3\12 oz.	82	285
Frankfurter (all beef)	1/8 lb.	550	110
Ham			
Fresh	1/4 lb.	37	260
Cured, butt	1/4 lb.	518	239
Cured, shank	1/4 lb.	336	155
Lamb			
Shoulder Chop (1)	½ lb.	72	422
Rib Chop (2)	½ lb.	68	398
Leg Roast	¼ lb.	41	246

Liver

Beef	31/2 oz.	86	325
Calf	31/2 oz.	131	436

Pork

Loin Chop	6 oz.	52	500
Spareribs (3 or 4)	31/2 oz.	51	360
Sausage (link or bulk)	31/2 oz.	740	140

Turkey

Turkey	31/2oz.	40	320

Veal

Cutlet	6 oz.	6	448
Loin Chop (1)	1/2 lb.	54	384
Rump Roast	¼ lb.	36	244

Fish

Clams (4 1g.,9 sm.)	31/2 oz.	36	235
Cod	31/2 oz.	70	382
Flounder or Sole	31/2 oz.	56	366
Lobster (1)			
Boiled, with			
2 tbsp. butter	3/4lb.	210	180
Oysters (5 to 8)			
Fresh	31/2 oz.	73	121
Frozen	31/2 oz.	380	210
Salmon (pink, canned)	31/2 oz.	387	361
Sardines (8) Canned, in oil)	31/2 oz.	510	560
Shrimp	31/2oz.	140	220
Tuna			
Canned, in oil	31/2 oz.	800	301
Canned, in water	31/2oz.	41	279

Snacks

Candy

Chocolate Creams	1 candy	1	15
Milk Chocolate	1 oz.	30	105

Ice Cream

Chocolate	½ pint	75	*

Vanilla	½ pint	82	210

Nuts

Cashews (roasted)	6-8	2	84
Peanuts (roasted)			
Salted	1 tbsp.	69	105
Unsalted	1 tbsp.	trace	111

Olives

Green	2 medium	312	7
Ripe	2 large	150	5
Potato Chips	5 chips	34	88
Pretzels (3 ring)	1 average	87	7

Dairy Products

Butter (salted)	1 pat	99	2
Butter (unsalted)	1 pat	1	2

Cheese

American, cheddar	1 oz.	197	23
American, processed	1 oz.	318	22
Cottage, creamed	31/2 oz.	229	85
Cream (heavy)	1 tbsp.	35	10
Egg	1 large	66	70
Milk (whole)	8 oz.	122	352
Oleomargarine (salted)	1 pat	99	2

Breads Cereals, Etc.

Bread

Rye 1 slice	128	33	56
White (enriched)	1 slice	117	20
Whole Wheat	1 slice	121	63
Corn Flakes	1 cup	165	40
Macaroni (enriched, cooked tender)	1 cup	1	85
Noodles (enriched, cooked)	1 cup	3	70

Oatmeal (cooked)	1 cup	1	
130			
Rice (white, dry)	¼ cup	3	45
Spaghetti (enriched, cooked tender)	1 cup	2	92
Waffles (enriched)	1 waffle	356	109
Wheat Germ	3 tbsp. 1	232	102

Beverages

Apple Juice	6 oz.	2	
187			
Beer	8 oz.	8	46
Coca-Cola	6 oz.	2	88
Coffee (brewed)	1 cup	3	149
Cranberry Cocktail	7 oz.	2	20
Ginger Ale	8 oz.	18	1
Orange Juice			
Canned	8 oz.	3	500
Fresh	8 oz.	3	496
Prune Juice	6 oz.	4	423
Tea	8 oz.	2	21

Fruits*

Apple	1 medium	1	165
Apricot			
Fresh	2-3	1	281
Canned (in syrup)	3 halves	1	234
Dried	17 halves	26	979
Banana	1 6-in.	1	370
Blueberries	1 cup	1	81
Cantaloupe	¼ melon	12	251

Cherries

Fresh	½ cup	2	191
Canned (in syrup)	½ cup	1	124

Dates

Fresh	10 medium	1	648
Dried (pitted)	1 cup (6 oz.)	2	1150
Fruit Cocktail	½ cup	5	161
Grapefruit	½ medium	1	135
Grapes	22 grapes	3	158
Orange	1 small	1	200

Peaches

Fresh	1 medium	1	202
Canned 2 halves,	2 tbsp. syrup	2	130

Pears

Fresh	½ pear	2	130
Canned 2 halves,	2 tbsp. syrup	1	84

Pineapple

Fresh	¾ cup	1	146
Canned	1 slice/syrup	1	96

Plums

Fresh	2 medium	2	299
Canned	3 medium, 2 tbsp. syrup	1	142

Prunes

Dried	10 large	8	694
Strawberries	10 large	1	164
Watermelon	½ cup	1	100

Vegetables*

Artichoke

Base and soft end of leaves	1 large bud	30	301

Asparagus

Fresh	2/3 cup	1	183
Canned	6 spears	271	191

Beans, baked	5/8 cup	2	704

Beans, green

Fresh	1 cup	5	189
Canned	1 cup	295	109

Beans, lima

Fresh	5/8 cup	1	422
Canned	½ cup	271	255
Frozen	5/8 cup	129	394

Beets

Fresh	½ cup	36	172
Canned	½ cup	196	138

Broccoli

Fresh	2/3 cup	10	267
Brussels Sprouts	6-7 medium	10	273

Cabbage

Raw, shredded	1 cup	20	233
Cooked	3/5 cup	14	163

Carrots

Raw	1 large	47	341
Cooked	2/3 cup	33	222
Canned	2/3 cup	236	120
Cauliflower	7/8 cup	9	206
Celery	1 outer, 3 inner stalks	63	170

Corn

Fresh	1 medium	ear trace	196
Canned	½ cup	196	81
Cucumber, pared	½ medium	3	80
Lettuce, iceberg	3 ½ oz.	9	264
Mushrooms (uncooked)	10 sm., 41g.	15	414

Vegetables*

Onions (uncooked)	1 medium	10	157

Peas

Fresh	2/3 cup	1	196
Canned	3/4 cup	236	96
Frozen	31/2oz.	115	135

Potatoes

Boiled (in skin)	1 medium	3	407
French Fried	10 pieces	3	427
Radishes	10 small	18	322
Sauerkraut	2/3 cup	747	140
Spinach	½ cup	45	291

Tomatoes

Raw	1 medium	4	366
Canned	1/2cup	130	217
Paste	31/2 oz.	38	888

NOW LET'S GO TO THE NEXT SECTION ON CALCIUM

Section 2: Calcium

Chapter 8: The Importance Of Calcium

Calcium occurs in the earth as limestone, calcium carbonate, as gypsum, or as apatite. It is always found combined with other elements. You will never find a pure calcium rock.

When these types of calcium compounds combine with water, they dissolve and form an alkaline solution. This is one of the reasons why you want to know as much about calcium, since it is one of the main elements that can make your body liquids alkaline.

One of the most important health programs you need to pursue is to move your body from an acid condition into an alkaline condition and calcium helps you do this.

When your body is maintained consistently in an acid condition, calcium is also consistently removed from your bones, which results in porous bones, or from tissue or organs causing degradation of those areas.

Calcium is the most abundant of the minerals in your body and it makes up 1.6% of your body weight or represents 40% of all of the minerals in your body. But, 99% of the calcium you have is located in your bones. The other 1% is distributed throughout your body, and it's involved in numerous structural and biochemical processes throughout your body.

Bone Loss

Bone loss starts around middle age. For women it increases during menopause. For men, bone loss is slow but steady starting from around 30. In bone loss there are normally no symptoms. But here are a few that stand out:

- ❖ Bone deformity or rickets
- ❖ Muscle and leg cramps
- ❖ Insomnia
- ❖ Growth retardation

Unfortunately, around 40% of women who live over 75 years will experience bone loss factures. Here are some reasons for low bone mass at any age.

- ❖ Diet that lacks daily use of fruits and vegetables
- ❖ Slender body or low weight
- ❖ Premature menopause
- ❖ Anorexia nervosa
- ❖ Extreme athletic training
- ❖ Lack of exercise or a sedentary lifestyle
- ❖ Excess eating or using various types of meat or protein, phosphorus, sodium, caffeine, wheat bran, and alcohol
- ❖ Smoking
- ❖ Excess use of sodas
- ❖ Use of corticosteroid medications
- ❖ Prolong bed rest or confined to a wheel chair

It has been found that if you lack a small drop in the required level of calcium in your body this deficiency will activate aging and many degenerative diseases. Even though calcium is a large atom, it chemically moves 10,000 times faster and is 10,000 times stronger than magnesium.

This gives calcium the ability to bind quickly and strongly with important biological molecules, which sustain life. This chemical flexibility gives calcium the honor of being called "the King of the Bioelements."

In this kindle e-book, you will discover why it has this name. Despite there is more calcium in the body than any other mineral, with exception of oxygen, calcium is not more important than the other minerals, since all work together and are needed in your body for maintaining life.

What we can say about calcium is that it is involved in more biochemical activities in your body than any other mineral, so that it is important to supply your body with a good amount of calcium. Your body will eliminate the excess calcium from your body as its natural behavior, even when it is in a super saturated form in your body liquids.

But when there is a deficiency of other minerals in your body that must balance with calcium, like sodium, excess calcium can react un-naturally, causing calcium crystalline deposits, which lead to pain and disease.

When your body lacks calcium and has weak or porous bones, calcium will deposit calcium crystalline stones in various places in your body as it tries to build up weak bones. A misconception is that if you have calcium deposits in the joints or tissue giving you pain, that you have too much calcium.

The truth is you do not have enough calcium, so the body tries to compensate for this by calcium deposit to build your bones back up.

Calcium is found in your blood, bone structure, tissue, muscles, lymph liquid, and in every body cell in your body. It is found in the lymph liquid outside and inside your cells. In the so called **Sodium – Potassium Pump** the mineral sodium moves out of the cell and moves potassium into the cell. When the inside of the cell has mostly potassium, the electrical charge inside the cell is less than the charge outside of the cell where sodium dominates. This condition attracts calcium to carry food nutrients into the cell and to perform in the cells various biochemical and bioelectrical reactions.

Calcium ions also play a major role in nerve stimulations and transmissions, muscle contractions and movements, and organ hormone secretions and many other biological functions. It is involved with your body's enzymes to produce energy.

Calcium ionic concentrations are the most regulated mineral in your blood plasma. Its ionic form is Ca^{++} and in this form its most important function is in nerve function. For nerve function, calcium keeps your nerves receptive to sodium ions which help to transmit brain impulses and information to various parts of the body, which regulate your body's activities.

In those cultures where drinking water had a high content of calcium, it was found that people's life span was 10 years or more than in western countries.

Kidneys

Your kidneys act as filters for your blood and they remove those nutrients or chemicals that your body no longer needs from your blood and this includes calcium. Excess calcium is routed to your bladder where it is expelled in your urine. If calcium is still needed, your kidneys will pass it into your blood to be reused by your body.

Most minerals and vitamins combine and react with calcium to produce the various body structures and chemicals that make up your body.

It was thought at one time that if you produced kidney stones that you needed to take less calcium. If you tend to form kidney stones, you will have increased calcium in your urine, but this is caused by your body pulling calcium out of your bones.

Because eating excess meat cause your body to excrete calcium it is recommended, for kidney stones, to eat less meat, increase the use of fruits and vegetables, and supplement with calcium citrate, magnesium, vitamin B6 and vitamin C.

You can take calcium citrate on an empty stomach. Most other supplements, you should take with meals.

Calcium Toxicity

Usually, there is no calcium toxicity, even when you take a large dose. There is some concern that people with a tendency toward kidney stones should avoid excess calcium, but these concerns have not been proven. Kidney stones are more related to diet and those people who favor an acid diet tend to form kidney stones. In an acid diet, calcium is active and depleted as it is used up neutralizing body acids.

Chapter 9: The Magic Of Calcium In Your Body

Here is a list of some of the important biochemical and bioelectrical functions of calcium in the body:

- ❖ Absorption of calcium
- ❖ Activity in cell function
- ❖ Maintaining an alkaline body
- ❖ Contributing to Saliva alkaline body test
- ❖ Needed Calcium foods

Adsorption of Calcium

Calcium is one of more difficult minerals to digest and to absorb through your intestinal walls. Various phosphates and other compounds (Phosphates are derived from phosphoric acid and when they combine with oxygen they become an organic phosphates, which have important biochemical activities in your body) found in red meat and sodas react with calcium to form a calcium phosphate precipitate. This prevents calcium from being absorbed and calcium is then excreted from your body.

However, when calcium comes in contact with the food substance of milk and various fruits and vegetables, it forms compounds that are easily absorbed.

For calcium to be absorbed into your body, it needs to have adequate vitamin D. Without Vitamin D, calcium cannot be absorbed into your blood stream. Vitamin D can be obtained from the sun and is critical in the amount of calcium absorption that occurs in your small intestine. This is why you need to get at least 20 minutes of sun every day. In some parts of the world less time is needed and in other parts more time is needed.

You can also get vitamin D from supplements. Some foods have it, but in very small quantities. When the sun's UV light hits your skin, fatty acids in your skin create vitamin D and **Inositol triphosphate, INSP-3**. This vitamin D finds its way into your intestinal wall where it assists calcium to move through your intestinal walls and into your blood stream.

Inositol triphosphate finds its way into every body cell. Its function is to release calcium from storage from within your cells, when insufficient calcium is not provided by your diet and supplements, or when insufficient vitamin D causes less calcium to be absorbed in the intestinal wall.

Inositol is obtained from foods such as fruits, vegetables, grains, and from liver, kidney and heart.

When there is insufficient calcium in the cell walls, because it got used up, the parathyroid hormone stimulated by deficiency of vitamin D activates the extraction of calcium from your bones. Once the bones become weaken, your body starts extracting calcium from proteins that regulate your cell functions. This results in a variety of aliment and disease symptoms.

Once in your blood stream, calcium is deposited in bones with the help of the hormone, calcitonin, released by parathyroid gland. Also, both Calcitonin and Inositol triphosphate regulate the storage and removal of calcium with in the cells.

The parathyroid gland is regulated by the pituitary gland, which is right behind the eyes. When you wear sunglasses this blocks the full spectrum UV light that is needed to regulate the pituitary gland, so that it can produce the hormones needed to regulate calcium in your cells.

Without adequate amounts of vitamin D, calcium will not be absorbed in proper amounts into your body and will just pass right through, excreted from your body.

Parathyroid – How it regulates calcium

The parathyroid is actively involved in maintaining your calcium blood levels. These levels are maintained to a very strict range. When your blood calcium levels drop, the parathyroid releases a hormone that directs the release of calcium from your bones and into your blood stream. And at the same time, it tells your kidneys not to excrete calcium into your urine.

Now, when you have excess calcium in your blood, the amount of the parathyroid hormone secreted is decreased. This causes the kidneys to expel more calcium into your urine. As all of this is happening, the parathyroid also releases a hormone called Calcitonin, which reduces the amount of calcium that is pull out of your bones.

Activity in cell function

Calcium is active in the process involving the Sodium-Potassium Pump in that it uses this pump to enter and exit from a cell. When it enters the cell, it brings in food nutrients to feed the cells. Once it releases these nutrients, it becomes a free ion. As these calcium ions build up in the cell, the voltage across the cell membrane will again reaches 70 millivolts. This sets the stage for nutrients and toxins in the cell to be pushed out of the cell and for other nutrients to enter the cell.

Maintaining an alkaline body

The fluid outside the cells is called extracellular fluid. This fluid is maintained at a pH of 7.4 by a calcium compound called calcium mono orthophosphate. This fluid is capable of neutralizing acids that comes out of the cells or arrive there from food that you have eaten. Sodium is also in the extracellular fluid and can neutralize acids, but it is needed in large quantities to maintain the Sodium-Potassium Pump cell activity. Wherever calcium is in the tissue, joints, blood, liquid or organs, it will neutralize acids. This process reduces damage to your tissues and elevates your body pH, making it more alkaline.

When you don't have enough calcium in your body, the cells will not have enough calcium to neutralize body acids and this will cause cell deterioration and will lead to various diseases. Keeping your body liquid alkaline or with a pH above 6.8 to 7.5 is what you should be working towards with any health program that you are working with. This can be done by using the right alkaline diet.

An alkaline diet helps you balance the level of acid and alkaline in all parts of your body. When you eat more acid foods, such as meat, butter, fats, carbohydrates, then your body needs to use up its alkaline stores to neutralize this acid, to prevent damage to your body's cells and tissue.

When you eat more alkaline foods than you need, you run the risk of not getting enough protein or carbohydrate and your pH can move above 7. 5 or 8.0 which can also lead to disease. You need a balance of certain foods to get your body pH in the range of 7.0

The saliva alkaline body test

In other kindle e-books, the saliva test has been discussed so that you can check its pH. This test is a strong indicator of whether your calcium ion level is sufficient. Here is a review.

When your Saliva pH is 7.0 to 7.5 it is considered alkaline and normal. When this is the case, your urine will be slightly acidic. When you lack ionic calcium, your pH will be 4.6 to 6.4 and your urine will be tend to be acidic.

Now here is important information. If you have physical ailments, your pH will be from 6.0 to 6.5. In this case, you should take around 2000 mg of calcium rather than 1000 mg. If your pH is below 6.0, mostly likely, you will have various disease symptoms. And, you should be taking around 3000 mg of calcium. Once you bring up your salivary pH, you can lower your calcium intake.

If your saliva tests show your pH to be below 6.0 then by taking more calcium supplements and by eating more fruits and vegetable during the day and especially in the evening, you can change your pH to 6.5 to 7.5

Keep in mind that the saliva test may not always be accurate, since the saliva pH can be influenced by food recently eaten. To get the most accurate reading, take the saliva test only after 2 hours of eating your last meal or snack. Also, bring saliva into your mouth 3 times and swallow, before taking the test. Take the test 3 times on 3 different days to make sure your readings are consistent.

In my kindle e-book called "Secret Diet And Nutrition Tips 1: Alkaline Body" I show you how you can change your body from 6.0 pH to 7.0 pH. In addition, in this e-book I show you how to do the saliva test properly so that you can get a good reading.

Simply changing your diet, taking vitamins, and mineral supplements when you eat, you can change your body's pH to the 7.0 to 7.5 level. When you do this, you will see a change in any physical aliment and disease that you might have. It will not occur instantly. You will need to keep this pH level for a few months.

Chapter 10: Illnesses Caused by Lack of Calcium

Calcium plays a major role in blood, cells, liver, kidney, and heart health. Calcium maintains blood pH to 7.40, solidifies bones, and helps heal scars, and fights scurvy and germs. It is present in cartilage, fluids, and tissue. It is useful for Indigestion, headaches, muscle pains, arthritis, ileitis, colitis, asthma. Lack of calcium creates problems, symptoms, and disease in the areas mentioned above.

The one thing to remember is that calcium from food sources does not contribute to arteriosclerosis, calcium deposits, increase blood pressure, and other illnesses.

Calcium is one of the main minerals that promote healing in bones, tissue, organs, brain and in all parts of the body. It is carried to various parts of the body through the blood vessels. When you lack calcium, the infected or weaken areas do not get repaired properly and disease sets in. Without the necessary calcium your body needs, blood coagulation is affected and excess bleeding can occur.

Sun Glasses

Sunlight is a necessary energy that helps to insure the absorptions of calcium. But sunlight also plays another important role in regulating calcium throughout your body.

Sunlight or full spectrum white light plays a major role in how the pituitary and pineal glands work. In the work place however, the lighting is artificial and this has a big impact on your long term health.

The use of sunglasses is quite popular and because of the many different sunglass tints that exist, people wearing them filter out the sunlight frequencies associated with that tint. Full spectrum light, like sun light, is necessary for proper function of the pituitary and pineal glands.

In the book, The Calcium Factor: The scientific Secret of Health And youth, 2000, Robert R. Barefoot & Carl J. Reich, M.D. say,

"When artificial full spectrum lighting is used, human calcium absorption increases, plants flourish and cows produce 15% more milk...Tinted glasses can eliminate a large percentage of the sun's spectrum and therefore affect you both physically and psychologically. Thus, full spectrum light plays a vital role in the maintenance of balanced hormonal system and is therefore indispensable in maintaining a balanced calcium serum."

Osteoporosis

Osteoporosis is the lack of calcium in the bone and it is estimated that over 30% of the older population will develop this condition. This is not a condition that results from old age, but a condition that comes from having an acid body for a long time.

Since the endocrine glands exert a great amount of control over calcium, the endocrine glands are put out of balance by sugar. This causes an imbalance in calcium and then shows up as cavities in your teeth.

It is the imbalance of calcium in your body that is the start of the development of chronic illnesses.

Menstrual Flow

Menstrual blood contains up to 40 times more calcium than regular blood. If you have excessive flow then you become depleted of calcium and iron. It is during this period that you should be eating kale, using liquid chlorophyll, and the many foods outlined in this e-book.

Without using a program that replaces your loss of calcium and iron during your periods, you open yourself to various diseases later on. For a diet that contains plenty of iron you can check out my kindle e-book called, "Quick and Easy Diet Cures 4 Iron Deficiency Anemia."

Teeth health

Your teeth are made up of calcium phosphate. They are kept healthy by your blood and the nutrients that you supply them. The external part of your teeth is protected by enamel, which is an extremely strong material. But, acids that form in your mouth, when sugar is eaten, create an excess of bacteria that can penetrate that enamel.

Having dental cavities is a sign of lack of calcium. When your body needs calcium and you have not provided enough in your diet or your calcium body stores are depleted, calcium is pulled out of your teeth and bones to bring your body back into calcium balance. This weakens the teeth and bacteria can penetrate the enamel causing tooth decay.

Arteriosclerosis

Arteriosclerosis is not caused by an excess of calcium. It is caused by the lack of sodium and chlorine salts. Calcium needs these salts to be properly used and to stay in solution and not precipitate out onto artery walls. It is needed so that artery walls don't become inflamed by acid damage and consequently need repair through plaque buildup.

Arteriosclerosis occurs when plaque builds up along the artery walls, which takes place over years. Eventually this plaque will narrow the arteries and cause reduced blood flow or blood flow blockage. Reduced blood flow will result in many different illnesses because cells will not be getting the proper oxygen and nutrition. Blockage will result in heart attacks.

Plaque is made up of phospholipids, collagen, triglycerides, fibrin mucopolysaccharides, cholesterol, heavy metals, proteins, muscle tissue, and debris, which are all bonded by calcium.

Plaque only occurs in arteries that deliver blood from the heart to your body and not in the veins that return blood to the heart. Cholesterol is not the cause of plaque, but even if it was it can be controlled by diet and not drugs. Eighty percent of the cholesterol in your body is created in the body and 20% of it comes from your diet. Your body uses cholesterol in every cell, in hormones, in nerve impulses, in the brain, and in the creation of vitamin D on your skin.

It is the cellular breakdown along the artery walls caused by acidity surrounding the wall tissue or free radical damage that prompts repair of that area and that is when plaque starts to build up on the wall.

Heart Disease

Calcium is central to good heart function. Since calcium ions are linked to proper cell function, any deterioration you have in your cell do to the lack of calcium will affect the cell structure of heart cells and to the cells of the arteries. This deterioration will lead to heart diseases.

In addition the ability of the heart to contract and expand is due to the ionization of calcium, Ca++.

Effects Of Excess Calcium

When your body has an excess of calcium, you will see external and internal boney growths. These growths can occur in any part of your body such as joints, tissue, organs, or muscle. The growths may appear as kidney stones or other precipitates that occur on your heels, shoulder joints, knee joints, or toe bones.

When you have excess calcium, you need to eat more fruits

and vegetables to get the natural absorbable vitamins and minerals, especially sodium. Sodium and calcium must always be in balance, lack of one or the other leads to a chemical imbalance, which results in various illnesses or diseases.

Illness or Conditions Due To Lack Of Calcium

Here some of the symptoms or conditions that occur when you lack calcium:

- tumors
- sores, abscesses, inflammations
- discharges
- deformed fingers, bones, hips cranial bones
- tooth decay
- undersized organs
- blood deficiencies
- back pain
- vomiting
- tuberculosis
- excess bleeding
- excess mucus discharge
- poor scar healing
- craving for salt
- bone softening
- swelling knuckles
- bronchial congestion
- wrinkled skin
- cystic goiter
- cyst formation
- nervous problems

There are so many illness and poor body conditions that occur when you lack calcium. You may have a few of these, but if they are consistent and they remain with you for a while, consider increasing your calcium intake.

Nervous Problems

Anxiety is supposed to help you when you are involved in stressful or life threating situation. Under these conditions your metabolism increases, muscles tighten, and you get a shot of adrenaline. When anxiety happens, you use up many minerals, including calcium. Under stressful conditions that last more than a day, it is wise to take a calcium supplement.

Back pain

Back pain is one of those conditions that when it occurs it can disable you and cause you to take a quick trip to emergency. When back pain is caused by strained muscles, stress, bad posture, in activity, or lack of exercise, one of the supplements recommend is calcium with magnesium. These minerals reduce muscle spasms, muscle tightness, and nerve irritation.

Taking a supplement that contains calcium, magnesium, and vitamin D daily, will help you to alleviate the long list of body conditions or illnesses. Just remember that calcium is a relaxer and nerve reliever.

Chapter 11: Eating The Best Calcium Foods

Even though you eat calcium foods, only around 25% of the calcium in this food will be absorbed by your body. But as a child or if you are pregnant, you may absorb up to 60%.

When cooking fruits or vegetables, you should use lower temperatures, when possible. When produce is heated to above 150 Fahrenheit at least 33% of the available calcium is lost.

Calcium and Milk

All milk that is pasteurized at high temperature is a low source of calcium. There is some milk that is pasteurized at 145 degrees Fahrenheit that are better sources of calcium. All milk that has been pasteurized or homogenized is acidic. The best milk source for calcium is raw goat milk and since it has not been heated it is alkaline in nature.

Despite the insistence from The Dairy Council that,

"Milk has been part of the diet for thousands of years. Despite the fact that milk is one of the most nutritionally complete foods available, there are many myths relating its consumption that blame milk and dairy foods for a variety of ailments. Many of these myths have been part of the folklore for centuries and are not founded on science."

There is tremendous amount of scientific papers and finding that milk should not be included in your diet, because of the illnesses it contributes too. But then again there are studies that show there is a decrease in heart and cancer in people that drink milk.

An article, In 1992 The New England Journal of Medicine pointed out that, "Consumption of cow's milk has been associated with insulin dependent diabetes..."

But this is also evidence that some milk should be drunk and that there are other sources of dairy products that can provide plenty of calcium for your diet, such as yogurt or cottage cheese.

Because of the tremendous activity of calcium in the body in relation to cell nutrition and it alkalizing effect, it is best to eat plenty of those vegetables and fruits that are high in calcium.

In his book, **Prescription for Natural Cures**, 2004, by James F. Balch, M.D. he says,

"It may surprise you to learn that countries where people drink the most milk are also those with the highest rates of osteoporosis. This may be due to the fact that lactose intolerance and casein allergy are very common and lead to mal-absorption. Also, calcium from cow's milk is not well absorbed, at a rate of 25 percent. Milk products lead to other health problems as well, so don't rely on them as source calcium. Unsweetened, cultured yogurt is an exception."

One way to eat your unsweetened yogurt is to add it to a blender and then add fruits like strawberries, pineapple, mango, bananas, and so on. To get additional sweetness, you can add some raw honey, since honey helps you to absorb calcium.

The British Medical Research Council made a 10 year study of 5000 men aged 45 to 59. In this study they found, "only 1 percent of those who regularly drank more than one-half liter of milk a day suffered heart attacks ... against 10 per cent of those who drank no milk at all."

In this study, researchers also found there was no difference whether they drank pure milk or skimmed, the benefits were still there.

There is still a lot of controversy about drinking milk for calcium. If you feel good drinking milk, then you should drink it. If you develop mucus or other symptoms, when you drink milk, then you should consider getting your calcium from other sources.

Where you can get calcium

One of the highest sources of calcium comes from **barley, green kale,** and **turnip greens**. You can get good calcium from cereals and grains.

Here is a list of foods highest in calcium:

- Seaweed – dulse, kelp, Irish moss, wakame, nori, sombu, agar
- Sardines with bones
- Tempeh, tofu
- Avocados, figs, prunes
- All dark greens, collard greens, spinach, kale,
- Unprocessed seeds and nuts – sesame seeds, grains, and nuts, almonds, walnuts
- Bone broth
- Cows, skimmed milk, cheese, cottage cheese, goat milk, yogurt
- Rice milk-calcium enriched
- Cabbage, cauliflower, celery, lemons, rhubarb
- Egg yolk, gelatin foods
- Fish, meat near the bone
- Whole wheat bread
- Beans, brown rice, lentils, millet, oats,
- Broccoli, Brussels sprouts, cauliflower
- Onions, parsnips, watercress
- Raw butter, gelatin, blackstrap molasses
- Coconut, raw cream, egg yolk
- Fish, meat near the bone, bone broth
- Natural cane sugar

The amount of calcium in certain foods

½ cup of wakame – sea vegetable gives 1700 mg
¼ cup of agar – sea vegetable gives 1000 mg
½ cup of nori – sea vegetable gives 600 mg
¼ cup of kombu – sea vegetable gives 500 mg
1 cup of tempeh gives 340 mg
8 oz. of calcium enriched rice milk give 300 mg
1 cup of almonds gives 300 mg
8 oz. of skim milk gives 302 mg
8 oz. of low fat yogurt gives 300 mg
1 oz. of Swiss cheese gives 272 mg
10 figs give 269 mg
½ cup of tofu gives 258 mg
½ cup of sesame seeds gives 250 mg
1 oz. of mozzarella cheese gives 183 mg
½ cup of boiled collards gives 179 mg
1 tablespoon of blackstrap molasses gives 172 mg
1 cup cottage cheese gives 126 mg
2 sardines in oil give 92 mg
¼ cup of walnuts gives 70 mg
1 cup of black beans or lentils gives 55 mg
½ cup of boiled mustard greens gives 52 mg
½ cup of boiled broccoli gives 36 mg

Dark Greens

The dark greens can be boiled instead of steamed and their taste is improved. Boiling them also does not cause them to reduce their nutritional value, since they has such high nutrition to begin with.

Meat

Limit the amount of meat you eat. Meat has 30 times more phosphorous than calcium. And, in the digestive tract, this phosphorous will cause the calcium to precipitate to form apatite, which is a form of a phosphorous calcium mineral crystal. It is apatite that is the substance that forms your bones. The result is that this calcium is not available to you and is excreted from your body.

Sugar

It has been found that there is 40% less calcium in white sugar as compared to raw sugar. Blackstrap molasses has 258 times more calcium as white sugar. Calcium and sugar attract each other. The more sugar you eat the more calcium is precipitated. The less body calcium you have the more tooth decay you will have.

Salt

Using excess salt in your food has been associated with bone loss. If you eat salt with your food, salt competes with calcium to get absorbed. The more salt is absorbed the less calcium is. Try using culinary herbs and chili sauces to flavor your food. If you like salty food, you could use them as a snack and not with your regular meals.

Nightshades

Foods like tomatoes, potatoes, eggplant, peppers and tobacco, which are considered nightshade foods.

In her book, Food and Healing, 1986, Annemarie Colbin points out that,

"In my own experience and that of some of my students, consuming nightshades on a dairy-free diet has resulted in a loss of calcium, evidenced by brittle nails, painful gums, and dental caries. Eliminating the nightshades, rather than increasing the dairy, solved the problem"

There are some foods that promote the excretion of calcium. We have indicated that eating excess meat can trap calcium and eliminate it from your body.

Foods high in oxalic acid also promote the removal of calcium from your body – spinach, cranberries, and rhubarb.

Wheat bran also limits the amount of calcium you absorb because to the phytic acid in its fiber. The phytic acid in wheat fiber has the ability to combine with calcium and limit its absorption in your body.

Other things that limit your calcium absorption are eating too many foods that contain phosphorus, drinking tea which contains tannins, lack of vitamin D, and having diarrhea.

Pumpkin Seeds

Shelled pumpkin seeds are a high source of zinc, magnesium, iron phosphorus, and calcium. You can eat a hand full every day.

Chapter 12: The Calcium Supplements You Need

Taking calcium supplements is a great idea, since you are probably not getting all of the calcium you need in your diet.

However, since calcium tends to interfere with the absorption of other minerals, it is best to also take a multivitamin that provides those other minerals.

What type of calcium supplements should you take? A good supplement is one that contains:

- Calcium 1000 – 1500 mg
- Magnesium 400 – 600 mg
- Vitamin D in Cholecalciferol form, called D3

So what are your daily requirements for calcium? Daily requirements for calcium are between 1000 to 1500mg. The type of supplement and the amount you take depends on your ability to absorb calcium. This is difficult to determine, so it is best to take the high end of calcium – 1500 mg.
Here are some minimum calcium supplementation requirements. Keep in mind that if you can get this amount in your food then you don't need to take calcium supplements.

Infants 7-12 months   270 mg
Children 4-8 years   800mg
Males 31-50   1000mg
Females 31-50   1000mg
Pregnant and lactating 1000mg

One of the best calcium supplements to use is Brazil Live Coral. It contains calcium, vitamin D, magnesium, and all of the trace minerals. It is in powder form so it is more absorbable. It contains the vitamin D you need to absorb the calcium.

But you also need to spend at least 20 to 30 minutes in the sun to get the natural vitamin D. It does not have to be in the direct sunlight, but it is better, if you can do it. Look on the internet for:

Brazil Live Coral

Also look for **Okinawa coral calcium** which is another good product.

Another excellent calcium supplement is called, **3-Way Calcium Complex™**. Look for this on the internet. It uses three different forms of calcium and includes other nutrients that help you absorb more of this calcium.

Calcium absorption

For calcium to be absorbed in the body, it is crucial to have adequate vitamin D in your body. Without Vitamin D, calcium cannot be absorbed into your body. Vitamin D can be obtained from the sun and from supplements. Be aware that wearing sunglasses can affect your health by not keeping your pituitary gland healthy.

It's the pituitary gland that tells the parathyroid to release hormones that help to regulate and absorb calcium. In addition to eating calcium foods, take Brazil Live Coral Calcium and also add vitamin D as a supplement to your diet, especially if you don't go out into sun every day.

Vitamin C

It is believed that by taking vitamin C with Calcium, you increase the absorption of calcium. A form of calcium that is already combined with vitamin C is called Calcium Ascorbate. This type of calcium is easily transported across the intestinal walls.

Chelated calcium

It is best to use calcium supplements in chelated form. What this means is that calcium is tied to an amino acid and this makes it easier for calcium to pass through your intestinal walls. Chelated calcium is more easily absorbed than calcium that is not chelated. Here are some of the types of calcium amino acid chelates you should look for and buy.

Calcium Alpha Keto Glucarate
Calcium ascorbate – a form of calcium that is tied to vitamin C
Calcium Lactate
Calcium Arginate
Calcium hydroxyapatite – the type of calcium found in your bones
Calcium Glycinate
Calcium Amino Acid Chelate
Calcium Caprylate
Calcium Malate
Calcium Gluconate
Calcium L-Aspartate
Calcium Lactate Gluconate
Calcium Lysinate
Calcium Orotate
Calcium Succinate

Tri calcium phosphate – the type of calcium in your bones
All of these amino acids tied to calcium can also be attached to the other minerals like magnesium and potassium. So you can find magnesium arginate or magnesium alginate or magnesium aspartate.

Honey

It has been found by the United States Department of Agriculture nutritionist Richard J. Wood that the glucose in honey can increase your absorption of calcium by up to 25%. It can also increase the absorption of zinc and magnesium.

Types of Calcium to avoid

Calcium Dolomite

Avoid using dolomite as a source of calcium, since it may not be absorbed properly by your body. Dolomite is a form of calcium carbonate and magnesium.

Calcium carbonate

Calcium carbonate is hard to absorb when the pH in your stomach is not at the proper level. If you low levels of stomach acid you will not be able to absorb this type of calcium.

Magnesium

Magnesium is usually found in calcium supplements because it is required for proper calcium metabolism. Magnesium has a role in the formation of bones. It has been found that when there is a decrease in blood magnesium that there is also a drop in blood calcium. The lack of magnesium in your body can increase the risk of osteoporosis.

Magnesium's absorption is enhanced by vitamin D just like calcium is. Magnesium is active in making sure that cells function properly by moving sodium and potassium in and out of the cells. Magnesium, just like calcium, is important for nerve and heart function. Many of the foods that are high in calcium are also high in magnesium.

Chapter 13: How Calcium Makes You Alkaline

In this chapter, you will discover how you can make your body more alkaline. Calcium in addition to other minerals is one of the main minerals that can help you do this. Keeping your body alkaline is one of the best ways to keep your body calcium levels in balance.

Minerals

Moving your body more toward alkalinity is what will give you the best curative effects of fruits. An alkaline body prevents your body from becoming ill and forming deadly diseases, like all kinds of joint problems, organ degradation, body pain, or even cancer. If you are already sick, then all of the chemicals inside fruits will help to revive you to better health. This is provided that your tissue damage has not gone beyond repair.

The minerals most important in changing and maintaining your body in an alkaline condition are sodium, potassium, chloride, calcium, phosphorus, magnesium, and sulfur.

Now, how your body can become alkaline might become a little confusing at first because of the terms used, but let's break this down into small parts. This process has been discussed in previous chapters, but this explanation gives more details. First we are going to be defining some terms so we can then start talking the same language.

Acid Binding

There are certain minerals that are called acid binding. And these are minerals, as mentioned earlier, are the most important ones in fruits, Sodium, potassium, chloride, calcium, phosphorus, magnesium, because they are acid binding.

What acid binding means is when you eat fruits with these minerals, your cells, after metabolism, create an alkaline ash. This ash will seek out acids in your body and bind with them to neutralize them.

Alkaline Ash

Now, that this alkaline forming ash has tied up an acid it is carried to the kidney where it is expelled as urine.

Different reactions can occur when an acid binding mineral, like say sodium, encounters an acid. Of course acids in the body are toxic, so the body has the priority of getting rid of them fast, since they can damage tissue and cause pain and disease.

Here is another path way of the acid binding mineral process when it combines with an acid.

The Acid Binding Mineral Process

When you eat acid binding food, the blood carries it to the cells where it is oxidized, digested, or metabolized. The result of this digestion is a carbonic acid salt of alkaline minerals, which reacts with body acids and binds with them. In this process, a weak carbonic acid is created. Now, this weak carbonic acid is taken by the blood into the lungs where it is released as carbon dioxide and water.

If not all the acid toxins are captured by acid binding matter, the remaining acids can be neutralized by body stores of alkaline minerals. If you don't have a good store of alkaline minerals, then these acids will remain in your body creating pain and disease.

But if you do have a good store of alkaline minerals, then these minerals will find these acids, capture them and bind with them. Then these acids are routed out through your urine or colon and out of your body.

So you can see the importance of getting a lot of alkaline minerals into your body. Without them, acids which do not get bonded to alkaline minerals would move back into body tissue and continue their body damage.

Alkaline Binding

Now, there are also minerals that become alkaline binding and these minerals are sulphur, chlorine, iodine, phosphorous, bromine, fluorine, copper, and silicon.

It is these minerals that when digested by a cell will produce an acid salt that will bind with alkaline minerals. These minerals will be excreted through your urine. When alkaline minerals are bonded to an acid salt, the alkaline mineral is removed from your body and your body becomes more acidic, the condition
you are trying to avoid. Although you need to eat both foods that are acid binding or alkaline binding, you want to eat more of the acid binding foods.

Keeping Healthy

One of the most important parts of health is keeping the lymph liquid around your cells clean and free of toxins. To do this you need provide alkaline minerals to occupy the lymph liquid and you need to remove the acids that accumulate in that liquid and in all parts of your body tissue. You can do this by detoxifying your body and providing alkaline minerals for your lymph liquid.

Body Detoxification

The highest priority of the body is to detoxify itself. One of the best way to help your body detoxify is to provide minerals that bind with acids that are in the cells, tissues, organs, and muscles. What these alkaline acid binding minerals do is to pull out the toxins that are dispersed throughout your body.

With the help of the liver which detoxifies the blood, the kidney that removes impurities from the blood and the lungs which removes the CO_2 which results from alkaline acid binding, your body is constantly detoxifying itself. But when it is over loaded with acid toxins from your lifestyle, a complete detox of your body becomes impossible.

Where do Acid Toxins Come From

So why is the body overloaded with toxins? Why can't the liver take care of these toxins? The liver has the function to remove acid wastes from natural food that is created by food digestion and cell metabolism. When it encounters acid wastes such as food enhancers, dyes, preservatives, pesticides, and the variety of additives, the liver does not always know how to break them down to make them harmless.

But your body does not give up so easily when it knows that the liver was not able to disintegrate food additives. What it does is it instructs calcium to bind with these toxic acids and to take them far away from the blood stream.

The result is that calcium binding with acid forms a deposit and this deposit can be placed in your teeth, your joints, and as bone spurs, which grow in your feet or shoulders, vertebra, or muscle tissue. These calcium deposits are very painful, and if you have ever experience them, you know how much.

Now, we have talked about acid toxins in the body that are brought in through food and the environment. But there is another factor that creates acid in the body and that is emotions that are occur through life stresses, like work pressures, divorce, friendship problems, martial issues, and other similar problems. These emotional problems create acidic molecules that embed themselves into your tissues just like food acids.

Body Organs

All body organs function to rid the body of acid waste or toxins. Lack of alkaline binding food causes deterioration of the function of these organs. Each organ has a specific function in the elimination and neutralization of acid wastes and it does this in conjunction with alkaline acid binding minerals.

Here is the list of the fruits that have the highest alkaline minerals and the ones that you should be eating. The percentage number next to them indicates the strength of the alkaline mineral and the closer to 100% the more effective it is as an acid binding fruit. However you should be eating all of these fruit not just the ones at the top of the list.

The percentage assigned to these fruits is based on fresh fruits that are organic and that they are not cooked, canned or mixed with sugar. If they are cook or otherwise processed in some fashion, this will reduce their effectiveness as an acid binding. However, they will still be effective in acid binding.

Acid Binding Fruits With Alkaline Minerals

In the list below are fruits with alkaline minerals that create an acid binding salt your body uses to neutralize acid wastes.

Fruits above 50% in value are more acid binding, which means they will more trap acid wastes.

Here is the list of fruits to eat in the order of priority.

1. **Fruits at 100% Acid Binding – Best fruits To Eat**
   Lemons, melons – any type, watermelon

2. **Fruits at 93% Acid Binding – Great fruits To Eat**
   Cantaloupes, dried dates, dried figs, limes, mango, papaya

3. **Fruits at 87% Acid Binding – Still Great Fruits To Eat** Kiwis, passion fruit, pineapples, raisins, umeboshi plums

4. **Fruits at 80% Acid Binding – Eat These Fruits** Apricots, avocados, bananas, fresh dates, fresh figs, currants, gooseberries grapes, grapefruits guavas, kumquats, nectarines, pears, persimmons, quince

5. **Fruits at 73% Acid Binding – Still Fruits To Eat** Apples, organs, peaches, pomegranate, raspberries, sour grapes, strawberries

6. **Fruits at 67 Acid Binding** – Still Neutralizes Acids Cherries

Fruits To Concentrate On

These are the fruits you should concentrate on eating. Also eat them every day, if possible, fresh lemon juice in the morning, watermelon during the day.

You can see which fruits give you the best acid binding effects and eating them 80% of your overall food intake will convert your body over to an Alkaline body.

NOW LET'S GO TO THE NEXT SECTION ON MAGNESIUM MAGIC

Section 3: Magnesium Magic

Chapter 14: Why You Need Magnesium

Half of the magnesium you have in your body is found in your bones and the other half is in your soft tissue. It is found in your skeletal muscles, liver, heart and pancreas.

Magnesium is considered a "forgotten mineral." Most people don't think about magnesium like they do calcium, potassium or iron. Almost 90% of the population may be short on magnesium, since it has been found that they only consume about 40% of the daily recommended requirement.

If you are short in magnesium, you may not show any symptoms, you may just ignore them, or you may attribute them to some other nutrient deficiency. However, moderate or severe magnesium deficiency results in malnutrition, loss of appetite, nausea, weakness, personality changes and arrhythmias.

Magnesium in Chlorophyll

Magnesium is a major mineral like sodium, calcium, and potassium. It is central to the food chain in that it holds a position in chlorophyll, the blood of plants. It appears in the center of the chlorophyll molecule. Chlorophyll is similar to the hemoglobin molecule except that at the center of the hemoglobin molecule is the mineral iron.

So, if you want to build your blood, drinking chlorophyll is one ways to do. It's the magnesium in the chlorophyll that also helps make white blood cells that fight infection and which combines with red blood cells.

When your body is low in hemoglobin, drinking chlorophyll will help increase the hemoglobin in your blood. Your body has the power to transmute or to transform magnesium into iron, which helps to make more hemoglobin. It does this through multiple chemical changes that start with oxygen.

Magnesium Requirements

The overall balance of minerals in your body's lymph liquids, outside your cells and inside your cells, determines your health. When your minerals are balanced similar to sea water, you will have better health.

The sea has a high level of magnesium, so that water inside your cells should also be high in magnesium, since magnesium is used to transport nutrients in and out of your cells. Magnesium is a major mineral that is needed in the right quantities, so that you can achieve maximum health.

Most people ignore the importance of magnesium. It is important to know what magnesium does in your body. You need to know what foods to eat to get the maximum magnesium in your body. You should know what symptoms you will have, when you don't get the proper amount of magnesium.

If you know how magnesium is regulated in your body, then you can help your body maintain and keep the amount that your body needs. Also, if you know what illnesses need more magnesium, you can help yourself get well.

Magnesium and Enzymes

Magnesium is involved in activating over 300 different enzymes and body chemicals. It helps to active the B vitamins. It works in protein synthesis, muscle excitability and helps to release energy. In your cells, it converts fat, carbohydrates, and protein into the energy your body needs. It helps to regulate blood sugar, nerve impulses, and electrical potential across cell walls. And, it tones brain blood vessels and keeps them relaxed and open, so that nutrients can get into your brain cells.

Magnesium and Bones

You will find magnesium mostly in your cells, in the mitochondria, which is the energy center of your cells. Magnesium regulated the absorption of calcium and maintains the construction of bones and teeth. Lack of magnesium can lead to brittle bones and osteoporosis. Your parathyroid gland also needs magnesium to regulate your blood calcium levels.

Magnesium is the third most important nutrient in building bones, after calcium and vitamin D. Half of all the magnesium in your body is found in your bones. When you lack magnesium, you are susceptible to forming calcium crystals in your bones and in other body locations.

Stress

If you are constantly under stress because of your job, you home life, or your regular life, then most likely, you will be low on magnesium. The same holds true if you stress your body physically by doing exercise and playing sports.

Chapter 15: The Magic of the Mineral Magnesium

"A mineral that relaxes the body – magnesium"

Like sodium, calcium, and potassium, magnesium also has a positive charge and is represented by the symbol, Mn+. Because of this, magnesium helps to make your body more alkaline. Your bones hold up to 60% of the body's magnesium, and the extracellular liquid contains around 1%.

Your body holds up to 3 oz. of magnesium. It is alkaline in nature and it is known as the "Relaxer", since helps to calm the nerves and muscle tissue. But, calming the nerves is also a matter of mind control and attitude. You can increase your life span, when you are calmer and have the proper amount of magnesium in your body.

In your body, magnesium takes the form of:

❖ Magnesium carbonate
❖ Magnesium silicate
❖ Magnesium chloride
❖ Magnesium sulphate (Epsom salt)
❖ Magnesium phosphate.

When you have plenty of magnesium in your body, you have good motion and can do many physical activities. Here is a list of what magnesium does in your body.

❖ Alkalinizes the body
❖ Produces laxative action
❖ Calms the nerves
❖ Keeps the body flexibly
❖ Influences glands
❖ Combats acids and toxins

- ❖ Eliminates poisons
- ❖ Prevents deposition of phosphates in joints
- ❖ Neutralizes phosphoric acid
- ❖ Promotes carbohydrate metabolism in the cells
- ❖ Helps produce and use body energy
- ❖ Helps in DNA and protein creation
- ❖ Assists Potassium and sodium cross cell membrane during Potassium – Sodium Pump action
- ❖ Regulates muscle movements
- ❖ Helps maintain calcium levels in the extracellular fluid

Magnesium does its work by reducing tension, relaxing your body, and improving bowel movements. It reduces nerve irritation by neutralizing the chemicals or by products that are created when your body is going through tense and irritable conditions.

Your body regulates the amount of magnesium it retains and stores by using the gastrointestinal tract, GI tract, and urinary system. If you need more magnesium in your body, the GI tract will absorb more in the small intestine. If your body has too much magnesium, the GI tract will excrete some of it and eliminate it through your stools.

Your kidneys are also involved in controlling the amount of magnesium your body retains. If magnesium levels fall, the kidneys closely control how much magnesium goes into your urine. Similarly, if the magnesium levels are too high, the kidneys will excrete more through your urine.

Regulation of Magnesium

Many things control how much magnesium and calcium you absorb. If magnesium in your body goes up, calcium stores will go down and if magnesium stores fall, then calcium body stores go up. Your stomach absorbs a lot of magnesium for hydrochloric acid production, HCl. When you take in food or calcium supplements, protein, vitamin D, or alcohol, your body needs more magnesium. And, caffeine, sugar, phosphorus, excess sodium, diuretics, and alcohol increase the loss of magnesium through urine.

You will increase the amount of magnesium you absorb, when you drink milk, because of the presence of lactose.

Magnesium as a laxative

Magnesium has natural laxative powers. When you eat foods that have magnesium your regularity improves. When magnesium is consumed and reaches your blood, some of it is transported into your colon walls. Where it softens your stools and helps to produce peristaltic action. For this reason fruits and vegetables that contain some or are high in magnesium promote regularity – yellow and winter squashes, grapefruits, apricots, oranges, peaches, and corn.

Chapter 16: The Best Magnesium Foods

Here is a list of the foods that you should eat to get plenty of magnesium:

Best foods with magnesium:

Rice bran, pumpkin seeds, wheat germ, sunflower seeds, sesame seeds, seaweed agar, cashews, hazelnuts, fermented soy products

Other great foods for magnesium:

Peanuts	leafy greens	seeds
Buckwheat	bananas	beet greens
Oats	avocados	black-eyed peas
Baked potato	with skins	blackstrap molasses
Cabbage,	dandelion	brown rice
Rice bran,	pomegranates	barley
Whole wheat	walnuts	mustard greens
Almonds	nuts	rye
Nettles	chestnuts	berries
Seafood	green leafy	vegetables
Dry beans and peas		meat

Chocolate

Many people crave chocolate. This may be because they are deficient in magnesium. Chocolate, especially cocoa, has a high concentration of magnesium. In one cup of unsweetened cocoa, you have 400 mg of magnesium and 2159 mg of potassium. It also has many other minerals, but in smaller quantity. Cocoa is also known for is high level of antioxidants.

To get the best benefits of cocoa, you need to eat chocolate that has at least 85% cocoa.

However when you eat chocolate candy, which has bittersweet chocolate, or semisweet baking chocolate, it has up to 65% sugar and a fat level of 20 – 35%. Cocoa has 2% sugar and has a fat level of up to 15%. Using unsweetened or bittersweet chocolate in cooking is ok, since its sugar level is 2 – 45%.

What is not good about chocolate is it is also high in caffeine and theobromine, which stimulate the adrenals that can lead to adrenal fatigue.

Yellow Cornmeal

Yellow cornmeal, high in magnesium, has excellent laxative powers. Use it 3 or 4 times a week and improve your regularity. Cornmeal, cooked slowly under low heat, can easily be use with children or adults that are constipated. Or, you can prepare raw corn soup by:

1 ½ cups raw corn off the cob
Vegetable broth to taste
2 bay leaves
1 ½ cup of raw milk, cream, or milk
Put all this into a blender and warm slightly

Calms the nerves

Magnesium is a relaxer of nerves. When you are tense, nervous, get irritated, or turn hot tempered, you develop ulcers, colitis, constipation, and colon spastic conditions. Magnesium will help to reduce or minimize these conditions. It enters the nerve fibers, with the help of albumin and water.

When you first take magnesium for nerves or for any other condition, you will have to use it for a month or more to see results. It takes that long and even longer for magnesium to fill your body reserves, so that it is available to constantly serve your body's needs.

If you have lower back problems, you need to have plenty of magnesium. When you are tense, any adjustments a chiropractor gives will go out of adjustment, when your body is low in magnesium. The adjustment will be made and your tense ligaments or muscles will pull back the adjustment to its previous position.

Magnesium is found in tendons, ligaments, tissue, joints, and nerves and helps them to relax and to maintain bones in position.

Cramps in your calves, at night, call for magnesium and calcium, which prevents the stiffening of tissue and muscle due to excess acids.

Alkalizes the body

Magnesium combines with acids, gases, waste, impurities, and toxins to clean your body and make your body more alkaline. Magnesium sulphate pulls toxic buildup and waste from your intestinal walls and eliminates them through your stools.

A good supply of magnesium is necessary to make your body alkaline and to combine with poisons and heavy metals. Magnesium has the ability to combine with poisons that create diseases. It combines with excess albumin, lead, phosphorus, chloride, antimony, ferrous sulphate, barium, muriatic acid, uric acid, urate acid, and ptomaine.

In the brain, magnesium combines with phosphoric by products that occur when you do excessive mental work.

Chapter 17: Magnesium - Deficiencies and Excesses

Deficiencies of Magnesium

When you become dehydrated, you lose magnesium. When you take calcium you will deplete your stores of magnesium. Drinking too much milk also will deplete your body's magnesium.

Young athletes that drink too much milk need to be careful, since they tend to lose magnesium. Retired and geriatric people should always take a magnesium supplement.

If you are taking diuretics of any kind, natural remedies or drugs, you will slowly lose your magnesium. The more diuretics you use the more magnesium you lose.

When you are deficient in magnesium, you are over sensitive about everything in your life. You are hyperactive, anxious, fidgety, energetic, mentally active, and industrious. There are so many symptoms when you are deficient in magnesium that it is hard to tell when you are deficient.

The more serious symptoms are muscle spasms and seizures. There is now some evidence that magnesium deficiency has an important role in many heart ailments. Dr. Alexander Heggtveit, at the University of Ottawa in Canada, found fatal attack victims with less magnesium than those that died of other causes.

You can have a magnesium deficiency after prolonged diarrhea and vomiting or with long term laxative and diuretic use. If you frequently drink too much alcohol then, you will be deficient in magnesium.

Elderly people are at high risk for magnesium deficiency, since they absorb it poorly. If they supplement with too much calcium or use too many drugs, this can deplete their magnesium body stores.

When you have a low level of magnesium, you will have an increase in calcium blood levels, which contribute to the formation of kidney stones. If the low levels continue, magnesium will be pulled out of the heart muscles, causing a disruption in its function.

When your blood levels of magnesium are low, your body takes magnesium that is stored in your tissues, which leads to muscle weakness, fatigue, irritability and nervousness.

Here is a list of symptoms you can have when you have a low level of magnesium.

* Head tremors
* Voice breaks or stammers
* Unclear conversations
* Feeling of doom
* Smelly feet
* Muscles are weak
* Constipation
* Poor kidney function
* Poor sleep
* Back pain
* Heart palpitations
* Eyelids twitch
* Osteoporosis
* High blood pressure
* Migraine headaches
* Appetite for acid food and drink
* Nausea
* Heavy head in morning
* Shoulder and neck muscles tense at night

Hypomagnesemia

A deficiency in magnesium is called Hypomagnesemia. This deficiency is when the amount of your body's magnesium falls below 1.8mEq/L. The unit mEq/L is a measure given to the amount of substance in a body per liter. This deficiency can occur when you:

- ❖ don't eat enough magnesium foods
- ❖ have poor absorption of magnesium in GI tract
- ❖ have excess magnesium loss in GI tract
- ❖ have excess magnesium loss in urinary tract – kidney
- ❖ use excess coffee, alcohol, sugar, and tobacco

Negative emotions also deplete magnesium that is in reserves and in intracellular liquid. If you constantly live these emotions below, then you will be short of magnesium:

Hatred, resentment, jealousy, quarrels, bitterness, temper outbursts, selfishness, greed fear, panic, worry, paranoia, overwork, over study, loss of love one.

Other symptoms you can have with low magnesium are:

- ❖ Cardiac arrhythmias
- ❖ Digoxin toxicity
- ❖ Laryngeal strid or Respiratory muscle weakness
- ❖ Seizures
- ❖ Arthritis deformans
- ❖ Poor elimination
- ❖ Over excitement
- ❖ Nervous headaches
- ❖ Ulcers
- ❖ Acute diarrhea
- ❖ Eyes tearing excessively or excess catarrh of eye lens
- ❖ Nosebleeds
- ❖ Sex brain nerve ends and nerve fiber irritation
- ❖ Decrease in electrical nerve impules
- ❖ Extreme colitis

- ❖ Urine retention
- ❖ Sleeplessness, fainting
- ❖ Hot temper, forgetfulness
- ❖ Drastic mood changes
- ❖ Increase in asthmatic attacks
- ❖ Free Radical Damage

When you are magnesium deficient, the body starts taking magnesium out of your cells. As you reduce cell magnesium, your muscles grow weak and nerves and muscles become highly irritable.

Free Radical Damage

Low levels of magnesium can magnify the damage caused by free radicals. It has also been seen that it can start the production of free radicals.

Excess of Magnesium

You can have excess magnesium in your body, when you eat an excess of magnesium foods, supplements, tonics or drugs. When you have an excess of magnesium in your body, the sedative effects of magnesium are intensified. Your memory decreases, you become less active, and do not have good reasoning skills. Your nerve endings become less sensitive and depressed and your perception and intelligence is decreased. You become less interested in life and you sleep more.

Hypermagnesemia

Excessive magnesium in your body is called Hypermagnesemia. This condition occurs when you have a magnesium level above 2.5 mEq/L. This condition is rare, since kidneys can quickly remove excess magnesium. But when it does occur, and the cause could be:

- ❖ Kidney dysfunction

- ❖ Addison's disease
- ❖ Adrenocortical insufficiency
- ❖ Excess use of antacids or laxatives
- ❖ Excess use of magnesium rich dialysate
- ❖ Excess use of TPN solutions
- ❖ Excess use of magnesium sulfate in treating seizures, or hypertension

Patellar Reflex

If your patellar reflex, the tapping just below the knee to see if the leg extension occurs, is absent, it's an indication that your magnesium level is 7 mEq/L or higher. This high level makes your nerves relax creating an absence of leg reflex in the patellar test.

Magnesium Laxative

Excess magnesium is quickly removed, from your body by the onset of diarrhea. But one of the issues is that you can develop an excess of magnesium when you use a large amount over-the-counter, drugstore products, for acid reflux or constipation. Overdose on magnesium is a rare occurrence.

Large amounts of magnesium can be toxic. You can end up with excess magnesium, if you have kidney disease or if your calcium body levels are low and your phosphorus intake is high.

Chapter 18: The Best Magnesium Supplements

Taking Magnesium Supplements

Do not take magnesium supplements if you have kidney weakness or disease. Also if you have heart problems, do not take more than 350 mg of magnesium. It is always safe to see your doctor about what dose you should take.

Fast Magnesium

If you have gut spasms or other body conditions where you need to receive magnesium fast, you can do it as follows:

Buy a Magnesium Chloride Solution 18%, Ecologic Formulas Brand, on the internet or at a health food store. Add 1-2 teaspoons to a glass of water and drink twice a day. The taste is not too good, but you will get magnesium into your body quickly.

It is estimated that a typical American diet provides only around 30% to 50% of the 500 mg of the daily requirements for magnesium. In addition, around 80% of the diets eaten in American are magnesium deficient.

Magnesium is easier to lose than other minerals and especially when you eat or take an increase in calcium. When you supplement with magnesium you should check that the supplement has equal amounts of magnesium and calcium. If it has more calcium, you will lose some magnesium. Or, it would be better to take magnesium as a separate supplement and taken when you don't take calcium.

Magnesium Citrate

Use a magnesium citrate supplement. Take this supplement after 8pm with vitamin C and pantothenic acid, since these three nutrients work together. Always take magnesium and all other minerals and trace minerals with tomato juice or apple juice or at meals with whole grapes, meat or digestive enzymes.

This provides acid to dissolve and absorb the magnesium quicker. You can also take it after 8pm or just before bedtime without any food.
.
There are other forms of magnesium that are also good, since they are tied to an amino acid or are so called "chelated." These are,

  ❖ Magnesium citrate
  ❖ Magnesium gluconate,
  ❖ Magnesium Aspartate
  ❖ Magnesium taurate
  ❖ Magnesium oxide – avoid using this type, because it is not as absorbable as the other types.

Magnesium and Calcium Supplements

Look for a combination supplement of calcium, magnesium, vitamin D and with a 1:1 ratio of calcium to magnesium. This type of ratio is hard to find, but you should be able to find it on the internet. Most ratios your will find are 2:1 with calcium being twice as much as magnesium.

Here is other some other magnesium combinations that you should consider, if you can't fine the supplements above:

Potassium- magnesium citrate
Magnesium citrate – potassium- taurine

Taking too much magnesium can cause diarrhea, lethargy or weakness. This mineral can also interfere with any antibiotic you might be taking, so it best not to supplement with it when taking antibiotics or even other drugs.

How Much Magnesium?

Some doctors and nutritionists say that, you should have twice as much magnesium as calcium in your supplement. This will insure that you will have strong bones. Most supplements that contain these minerals are of the opposite ratio; they have twice as much calcium as magnesium. But, taking a supplement with a 1:1 ratio should be where you can start.

Daily magnesium supplementation is:

Children to 14 years, 270 mg
Males 15 and older, 500 mg
Males 51 years and older 600 mg
Females 15 and older, 300 mg
Females 51 years and older 550 mg

In some cases for adults up to 1200 mg is recommended. Over dosing is very hard with magnesium, since the kidney and the colon will excrete the excess. If you start to exhibit signs of diarrhea or body weakness, back off on the amount you are taking.

Vitamin D

You need the proper levels of magnesium to activate the vitamin D your body needs. If you have a magnesium deficiency, then you will have lower levels of vitamin D. Make sure you have the Vitamin D3 type of supplement.

B vitamins

When you take Vitamin B6, you improve the intake of magnesium into your cells. You can supplement with a vitamin B 50 or 100 to get the needed B vitamins.

Copper

Because magnesium is easily lost in the urine, when you are dehydrated, you can take 3 mg of copper and this will stop the loss of magnesium in your urine.

Over The Counter Magnesium Products

Magnesium toxicity can occur with individuals with kidney failure. Toxicity effects have been found in some individuals that use laxative such as Epsom salts, magnesium sulfate and milk of magnesia, or magnesium hydroxide. These laxatives are typically used at 3,000 to 5,000 mg per day. Toxic effects have been found when these laxatives are used at 9,000 mg per day.

If you have a deficiency of magnesium, it will take around 6 months of magnesium supplementation to get your body back to normal levels of magnesium. Your body uses magnesium every day, so you need to supply it with this amount every day. Any excess can go to neutralize acids. Then if still have some left over, this will go to various body areas to be store.

Chapter 19: Illnesses Eliminated With Magnesium

There are certain illnesses that you can reduce, eliminate and even cure, if you increase your intake of magnesium. Some of these illnesses are caused by the lack of magnesium.

These illnesses are:

- ❖ Cardiovascular
- ❖ Chronic fatigue syndrome
- ❖ Kidney stones
- ❖ Muscle cramps
- ❖ Preeclampsia – during pregnancy
- ❖ Osteoporosis
- ❖ PMS symptoms
- ❖ Migraines
- ❖ Respiratory disease
- ❖ Alzheimer's disease
- ❖ Back problems
- ❖ Free Radicals
- ❖ Migraines
- ❖ Digestive Problems
- ❖ Eye problems
- ❖ Constipation

Cardiovascular

Having a low level of magnesium can result in more blood clots. It has been found that women that use oral contraceptive have lower levels of magnesium. This is the reason why there is a higher occurrence of thrombosis in women that use these contraceptives.

A deficiency of magnesium can damage the arteries in the heart, which results in plaque buildup. High blood pressure is also associated with a magnesium deficiency. There is a tendency for those with diabetes and low magnesium to have more cardiovascular issues.

So keep your levels of magnesium high by eating and supplementing with the suggestions given here. Magnesium helps to reduce the possibility of you having a heart attack, stroke, angina, or heart surgery. Eating nuts of various kinds every work day will help you stop heart attacks.

Kidney Stones

If you have kidney stones, you can get rid of them by using 1000 mg of magnesium citrate and 100 mg of B6. If you just want to make sure you don't accumulate stones, you can use this supplement combination on occasion for a week. Kidney stones are a combination of calcium and oxalic acid. When these two combine in the kidney they form calcium oxalate crystals.

To minimize the amount of oxalic acid you have in your body, avoid eating cooked spinach or other green tops. Eat them raw when possible.

Muscle Cramps

Magnesium helps to relax muscle and without it you are prone to muscle cramps. When calcium moves into muscle tissue, your muscles will contract. When calcium leaves the muscles, and magnesium moves into your muscles, your muscles will relax. Excess deficiency of magnesium leads to muscle spasms, tremors, and convulsions. If you have leg cramps at night, take a combination of calcium, magnesium, and vitamin D. This will put an end to these cramps. Take this supplement just before bedtime.

Osteoporosis

To have strong bones and teeth you need minerals. It's

calcium that makes bones strong in conjunction with other minerals such as phosphorous, magnesium, strontium, silica, zinc, copper, and boron. Magnesium is definitely needed to prevent osteoporosis.

PMS symptoms

There are some women that crave chocolate before their period or who have PMS. It is known that magnesium helps resolve the symptoms of PMS, since it is involved in the production of progesterone. A lack of magnesium can produce decreased progesterone levels resulting in PMS symptoms.

It's better to avoid chocolate, since it creates adrenal fatigue. It is better to eat those foods that are high in magnesium or to take 400 mg of magnesium citrate. Take this magnesium with some vitamin C and B6 just before bedtime. Magnesium is absorbed better after 8pm. This combination of nutrients will help to reduce the intensity and duration of PMS.

Pregnancy

Magnesium has a powerful influence in the prevention of pregnancy complication, such as prematurity and intrauterine growth retardation.

Migraines

There are studies that show magnesium can prevent or relieve migraines. By using high doses of 1000 mg or more, magnesium was shown to be just as effective as established drugs, such as flunarizine and amitriptyline.

Respiratory Disease

Magnesium has been found to be helpful in respiratory disease such as bronchitis and asthma. Eat those foods that are high in magnesium, but you need to be aware of those foods that you might be allergic to, which aggravate your respiratory condition.

Alzheimer's Disease

Having a low level of magnesium and calcium in your body opens you up to toxic aluminum deposit in your brain nerve cells. When you have these low levels of these minerals, your body will accept the use of other minerals in their place. So if you also have an excess of aluminum, your body will use it in place of magnesium or calcium and when these minerals reach your brain they deposit in your brain cells.

The result is that you have the onset of senility or you develop Alzheimer's. Under these conditions, zinc is the recommend mineral to prevent senile changes in your brain.

Magnesium is involved in keeping your brain cells alive. It does this by reducing the negative effects of less blood flow to the brain and by insuring that nutrients reach your brain cells. It also prevents the buildup of calcium in your brain cells, which is associated with Alzheimer's.

Back Problems

Magnesium will help you build a strong straight back. It aids in the inter-vertebral structure. It is in this structure where magnesium is stored. It is also stored in the colon. If the vertebral structure and colon don't get enough magnesium, they will not function properly.

Free Radicals

It has been seen by researchers that low levels of magnesium give way to free radical formation thus exposing cells to more radical attack.

Migraines

It has been found that 50% of people with migraines have

magnesium deficiency. You can get some relief by taking 400+ mg of magnesium daily with meals.

Digestive Problems

If you have stomach problems such as vomiting, cramps, indigestion, flatulence, stomach pain, or constipation, all this could be related to low levels of magnesium.

Eye problems

If you are diabetic, you will want to keep high levels of blood magnesium. If you do, you are less likely to develop diabetic retinopathy. In addition, if you have glaucoma, it will lessen the effects of this condition.

Constipation

Magnesium is hydrophilic and likes water. In your colon it will draw water and make your stools soft. Magnesium is used in many over-the-counter laxatives. Using these laxative, gives you high levels of magnesium salts. If you are deficient in magnesium, you will have constipation.

Sweaty Hands

Have you ever shaked hands with someone that has sweaty hands or that has excess body order? Aside from not showering frequently, this person may be deficient in magnesium. The use of liquid chlorophyll will help reduce the body order.

Chapter 20: Final Magnesium Comments

In your cells, tissues, muscles, and nerves, magnesium neutralizes acids, toxic matter, and wastes that are created when you become anxious, nervous, hot tempered, over excited, or overworked. It helps to neutralize those acids that come from eating too much acid food. Use magnesium foods and supplements to help get your body alkaline.

When you eat a lot of meat and other acid foods with little vegetables, you will deplete your stores of magnesium and you will need to use all the information listed in this book to restore your magnesium body levels. Magnesium is known as the "Relaxer" since it calms your nervous and muscular system.

You can have an under or over supply of magnesium in your body. Your kidney and colon are responsible for maintaining the proper magnesium balance in your body. It will excrete excessive magnesium into your urine or it will stop excreting it when your body supplies are low. And, with under supplies, magnesium will be pulled out of your cells to satisfy your body's needs. When it does this your body will be acidic and prone to disease.

Eat Magnesium Foods

Eat magnesium foods daily. Use seeds in your smoothies and nuts as midday snacks. Eat a variety of vegetables. Choosing 4 or 5 vegetable properly can give you plenty of all the minerals you need. However, by choosing a variety of fruits and vegetables, you get certain nutrients and antioxidants that are only available in each fruit or vegetable.

Magnesium Supplements

When you buy a magnesium supplement it is best to buy it with calcium and vitamin D. Calcium needs magnesium and vitamin D to complete its digestion and absorption into your body. Choose those supplements that are tied to an amino acid, like Magnesium Citrate. This allows this mineral to be pulled through your intestinal wall easier and faster. Look for a magnesium supplement that has just as much magnesium as calcium, 1:1.

If you have a lot of anxiety and stress in your life you will need to take up to 1000 mg of magnesium. Stress uses up a lot of magnesium.

Look at the list of illnesses and body conditions listed in the previous chapters and see if you have some of these symptoms or diseases. If so, then you too should be taking up to 1000 mg of magnesium. If you have issues with your kidney or heart, then talk to your doctor about how much magnesium you should take.

Excess Magnesium

If you take too much magnesium, you will get diarrhea. Just back off on the amount you are taking, until your diarrhea goes away.

Chapter 21: About the Author With Resources

Rudy Silva is a natural consultant nutritionist educated in the United State in Nutrition and Physics. He is a graduate from the San Jose State University in California. He is author of 30 other e-books on natural remedies. He has authored a newsletter in natural remedies for over 4 years. He has many websites promoting special recommended products and information.

Resource page

Here are some of the other kindle e-books about natural remedies that have been written by this author. You can see the entire list at:

http://tinyurl.com/b2f7wd3

Acne Remedies
Best natural acne treatments: Acne facial

Constipation Remedies
Best Constipated Women Natural Cures
How To Relieve Constipation With Fruits

Essential Fatty Acids
Taking The Mystery Out Of Essential Fatty acids
Amazing Fish Oil Benefits Revealed

Nutrition Remedies
Updated Version - Secret Diet And Nutrition
Secret Healthy Fruit Practices Revealed
Fast Healing Juice Nutrition Therapy: Nutrition Tips 3
Fantastic Alkaline Fruit Benefits Revealed

Calcium (Discover How To Use Calcium To Avoid Devastating Diseases)
Magnesium Nutrition Revealed
Best Nutrition Health Practices
Potassium Health Secrets Revealed
Phosphorus, The Best Brain Food
A Sodium Diet (What You Must Know About Sodium)
Vegetables and Vegetable Juice Cures

Stomach Remedies
Acid Reflux: Fast and Easy Cures For Acid Reflux
Asthma Treatment Cures With Remedies
How To Do Natural Colon Cleansing
Gastrointestinal Digestion Secrets Revealed

Misc Remedies
Natural Hair Loss Treatment: Women And Men
Effective Natural Hemorrhoids Treatment
Iron Deficiency Anemia
Secrets To Understanding Behavior
Fast Acting Ear Infection Remedies
Best Impotence Health Diet
What Is A Hiatus Hernia
Best Varicose Vein Treatments?

Men's Health
Best Impotence Health Diet

Weight loss
Ten (10) Day Quick Success Weight Loss Program: A new approach to losing weight by changing your eating habits for life

To see all of the kindle books written by this author, go to this the Authors Profile Page or this URL:

http://tinyurl.com/b2f7wd3

If you need support or want to promote any of his e-books, please contact him at rss41@yahoo.com and expect a reply within 24 hours. He looks forward to hearing from you and is happy to help you understand his material on natural and nutritional health.

Give A Review

And, don't for get to give a review for this e-book at Amazon so that others can gain the benefits of what is in this e-book.

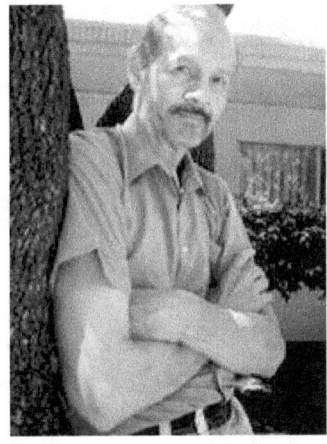

To you, for losing weight, creating better health and more happiness in your life,

Rudy S Silva

www.ingramcontent.com/pod-product-compliance
Lightning Source LLC
Chambersburg PA
CBHW070539290526
45790CB00002B/560